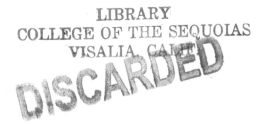

NOTES ON NURSING:

WHAT IT IS, AND WHAT IT IS NOT.

BY
FLORENCE NIGHTINGALE

With an Introduction by
Barbara Stevens Barnum

and Commentaries by
Contemporary Nursing Leaders

COMMEMORATIVE EDITION

J. B. LIPPINCOTT COMPANY
Philadelphia

Editor: David P. Carroll
Editorial Assistant: Patty L. Shear
Project Editor: Mary Rose Muccie
Production Manager: Helen Ewan
Production Coordinator: Kathryn Rule
Designer: Susan Hermansen

3 5 6 4

CIP data is available.

ISBN 0-397-55007-3

Photo of Florence Nightingale on page iv courtesy of the Hospital and Nursing Archive, University of Michigan, Ann Arbor, Michigan.

Photo of Florence Nightingale on page 2 courtesy of the Center for the Study of the History of Nursing, School of Nursing, University of Pennsylvania, Philadelphia, Pennsylvania.

Table of Contents

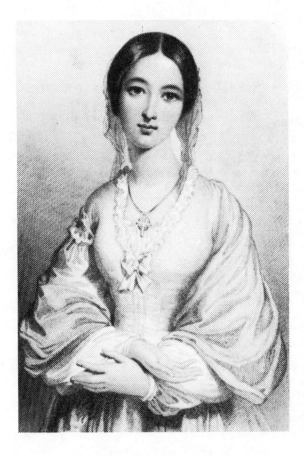

INTRODUCTION.

Lippincott is pleased to bring you this special reissue of Florence Nightingale's *Notes on Nursing.* In addition to Nightingale's original words, exactly as they appeared in the first printing, this centennial edition contains the thoughts of some of our most esteemed nurse–theorists and thinkers as they reflect on Nightingale. We asked each nurse–theorist to consider how Nightingale's work affected—or didn't affect—her own theory. We invited other nursing leaders to give us any thoughts about Nightingale they wanted to share. Hence, this book combines the thoughts of the founder of modern nursing with the thoughts of some of today's leaders.

When reading the contributions from the nurse–theorists, whose work represents a broad spectrum of theory, I was impressed by the fact that Nightingale had something to offer every one. Perhaps the true mark of greatness is the diversity of one's followers, and in this Nightingale excels.

As I reread *Notes on Nursing,* I couldn't help but think about the settings of Nightingale's greatest achievements—in Scutari, in the midst of war, and then the many years she spent as an invalid at home. These two environments, so different from each other, gave Nightingale the perfect settings for her work. The opportunities offered by the Crimean War seem more obvious—there were pressing needs for attention on all sides—yet her invalidism offered a unique advantage. As an invalid, Nightingale was removed from the tiring demands of everyday life. And few could resist the requests of one whose own health seemed sacrificed to her cause. The advantages of invalidism are sometimes overlooked by Nightingale's biographers, but in some ways that limitation was a singular advantage. Nightingale's invalidism gave her the freedom from other obligations; it allowed her to concentrate on her work. What modern mother juggling career, family, and home would fail to recognize the advantage of such time out? These and other thoughts about Nightingale's life and achievements are sure to be stimulated by the brief but insightful biography provided for this special edition by Nightingale scholar Dr. Constance B. Schuyler. I think you'll enjoy the refresher.

What was it that enabled Nightingale to stimulate the development of a profession, change the health and lives of so many, and still draw criticism and praise from a generation of nurses as far removed in time as our own? Enjoy the thrill of rereading Nightingale as well as the joy of learning how such a rereading stimulated the minds of many of our nursing leaders.

Barbara Stevens Barnum

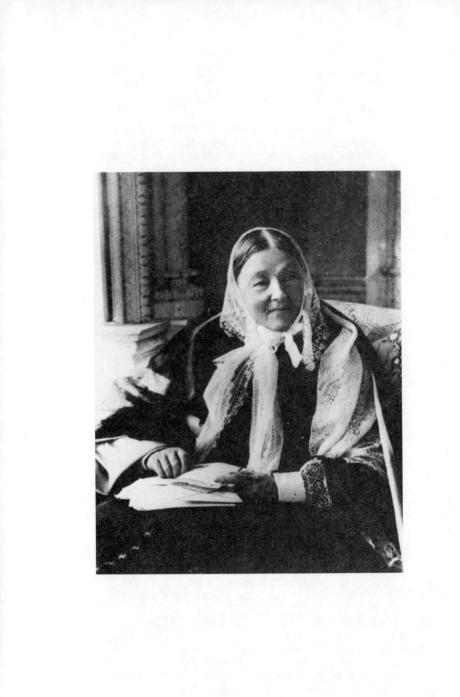

FLORENCE NIGHTINGALE.

Constance B. Schuyler

On August 15, 1910, two days after Florence Nightingale's death, *The New York Times* stated, "Few lives have been more useful or more inspiring than hers." A year later a memorial was established for her in London. The Lord Mayor of London remarked, "This memorial was intended to commemorate the work of one who was perhaps the greatest Englishwoman who ever lived." These accolades from both sides of the ocean may sound exaggerated but they are valid. Nightingale is one of the greatest reformers of modern times. Yet few today are aware of her genius, her commitment, or her extraordinary accomplishments.

Florence was the second child of William and Frances Nightingale. She was born on May 12, 1820, in Florence, while her parents were on an extended vacation in Italy. Her sister, Frances Parthenope, had been born a year earlier in Naples. Their father was independently wealthy. Having failed in his one attempt to be elected to a seat in Parliament, he turned his full attention to the education of his daughters. Florence was more interested in intellectual pursuits than her sister, and she became the focus of Mr. Nightingale's educative efforts. The family lived in comfortable circumstances at Lea Hurst and Embley Park in England, where numerous relatives were frequent visitors.

In spite of her family's wealth, Florence showed an early concern for the sufferings of others. She was a sensitive, introspective, and somewhat morbid child who never seemed to be satisfied with herself. She had a perfectionist nature, and as she matured, felt driven to improve herself and her world. She developed into a deeply religious person and came to believe that she

Constance B. Schuyler, Ed.D., R.N., is Associate Dean of Academic Affairs, Wagner College, Staten Island, New York.

was personally called by God to help others. She recorded her calls from God in her notes from childhood on. She believed that God wanted her to work with Him to improve the well-being of mankind. She wrote, "The highest honor is to be God's servant and fellow worker."

Nightingale was driven throughout her life by an intense commitment to help humanity. She had no time for pleasure, marriage, or social amenities. She devoted her life to the mission of improving the misery and unhealthy living conditions of people all over the world. Two powerful forces shaped her life: ideals and a need to act on those ideals. She commented, "The most practical way of living for God is not merely thinking about Ideals, but doing and suffering for Ideals." Her commitment to carry out her religious ideals helped her achieve far-reaching reforms in her lifetime.

Nightingale was a brilliant woman and an accomplished statistician. She used statistics to demonstrate the need for improvements in sanitation and health care. Her ability to use scientific research to demonstrate the need for reforms helped her immensely in her mission to improve people's lives. She accomplished reforms in health and sanitation in the British Army, in civilian hospitals, in workhouses, and in homes in England and other parts of the world. She worked to change the laws in England and India to improve the health of their populations, and she created the profession of nursing.

When she was young, Nightingale did not have a clear understanding of what her calling was to be. In 1844, she received what she felt was a definitive call; it was a call to do hospital work. She later wrote, "Since I was 24 there never was any vagueness in my plans as to where God's work was for me." She was held back from her calling for nine more years, however. She carried on a bitter struggle to break out of the restrictions of her family and society, which prohibited her, as a lady, from taking up nursing. Nightingale persevered in her efforts to pursue nursing and finally gained some education in this art. She began her career in 1853, in London, as the superintendent of The Institution for the Care of Sick Gentlewomen.

After one year in this position she was asked by Sidney Herbert, the Secretary for War, to take command of a group of women who were going to Scutari in Turkey to care for the wounded soldiers of the Crimean War. When Nightingale arrived in Scutari, conditions in the hospital were so terrible that almost one half of the soldiers admitted died. Nightingale's reform of the nursing care of the British soldiers during the Crimean War is probably her most well-known achievement. She not only nursed the sick and wounded, she also accomplished the enormous task of cleaning up the grossly unsanitary conditions in the military hospitals of the Crimean theatre.

When Nightingale arrived at the Barrack Hospital in Scutari, she calculated that there were four miles of mattresses with sick and wounded men lying on them. There was liquid filth from clogged sewers on the floors, and cases of cholera and typhus abounded. Nightingale had to deal with hostile doctors and administrators to obtain permission to establish sanitary measures and give the soldiers the necessary care. When she found that these measures were not effective, she wrote numerous letters to government officials in London urging them to investigate the structure and plumbing of the hospitals. Her pressure finally resulted in the dispatch of a Sanitary Commission, which went on to find major defects in the system of health care and sanitation in the hospitals. The Commission mandated action to clean up the situation, and the mortality rate dropped.

When the war was over in 1856, Nightingale came home unobtrusively on a mail steamer. She was weak from illness and overwork, yet she was so devastated by the horrible conditions she had witnessed that she was determined to prevent them from happening again. Because of her success in the army hospitals, the country adored her. They lauded her in books and poems and raised £45,000 for the Nightingale Fund to create a school for nurses.

In addition to the public support present already, Nightingale was able to gain more support for reforms through persuasive written and spoken pleas. Years ahead of her time in statistical analysis, she compiled statistical data on health conditions in the Army and used these data to write reports on areas that needed reforming. Early in 1857 she compiled data and wrote a report of nearly 1000 pages entitled *Notes Affecting the Health, Efficiency, and Hospital Administration of the British Army.* This report, which took six months to write, proved conclusively that more men died from the unsanitary conditions in the army hospitals during the war than from bullets on the battlefield. It also showed that sanitary conditions were so poor in army living quarters, even in peacetime, that the mortality rate of soldiers living in barracks was double that of civilians.

Nightingale wrote this report to help convince the Secretary for War, Lord Panmure, of the necessity of establishing a Royal Commission to investigate and reform the health administration of the Army. Her report was not officially published, but she had it copied and distributed to influential people at her own expense. Nightingale was the recognized leader of the reform group and she used her powers of persuasion to influence the appointment of a Royal Commission with members who would be sympathetic to her cause.

The Commission was finally formed with men who, but for one exception, solidly backed Nightingale. She persuaded Sidney Herbert to take on the chairmanship, but it was Nightingale who masterminded the Commission's inquiry. She determined the facts that were presented to demonstrate the need for reform. As each branch of the inquiry came up, she sent information to Herbert and suggested the best available witnesses. She even prepared some of the briefs for examination and cross-examination. The reform group referred to her as their Commander-in-Chief.

In August 1857 the inquiry was over and Herbert wrote the report with Nightingale's assistance. Their plan of action was that four subcommissions should be appointed to carry out the details of reform. Herbert outlined the plan to Lord Panmure. The subcommissions were to:

Put the barracks in sanitary order;
Organize a Statistical Department of the Army;
Institute an Army Medical School; and
Reconstruct the Army Medical Department.

Panmure agreed to creation of the subcommissions but procrastinated in taking any action. He was being pressured by both the pro-reform group and the anti-reform element led by Benjamin Hawes, the Under Secretary for War. Panmure's typical reaction was to avoid decision. In private, Nightingale angrily accused Panmure of defeating all her reforms. She complained to a friend, "We have seen terrible things in the last three years, but nothing to my mind so terrible as Panmure's unmanly and stupid indifference."

Nightingale was near exhaustion. She had pushed herself unremittingly in writing reports and setting up the Royal Commission. She had also been working with the Nightingale Fund to develop a school for nurses. Her health had deteriorated from the strain of overwork. She had become an invalid, but her work continued. She wrote, "Only do the work, do the thing." Her Aunt Mai left her own family and came to stay with her. Aunt Mai cared for her and protected her from all intrusions on her time, including her mother and sister, whom Nightingale considered especially obstructive to her work.

For several years Nightingale believed that her death was imminent so she pushed herself to finish her mission before it was too late. She was so intent on accomplishing her goal that she demanded a great deal from anyone who was willing to help her. Two men who were especially devoted to her and to her cause, Sidney Herbert and Arthur Clough, strained themselves to help her achieve her goal. Both men suffered from debilitating illnesses but continued to work for her in spite of their deteriorating health until the times of their deaths.

Herbert worked in an official capacity to carry out her reforms and Clough worked as her secretary. Herbert had sent Nightingale to Scutari, and because of her experiences there, he was totally committed to her efforts to reform the health administration of the Army. He assumed the chairmanship of her four subcommissions for reform. He was also chairman of the Royal Commission on Health of the Army in India and a member of the House of Commons. Clough's only official job for her was in connection with the Nightingale Fund, but he worked tirelessly as her private secretary. Clough's biographer, Robindra Biswas, states that no task was too menial for him as he worked against the clock to help Florence finish her work before she died.

By the end of 1859, Nightingale began to see that the very organization of the War Office's administration system was holding up the achievement of reform. She decided that the War Office itself must be reorganized, and given his superior organizing ability, Herbert was the only man who could do it. She pinned all her hopes on Herbert, but she was to be disappointed—he was dying of a kidney disease. He worked for another year preparing the scheme for the reorganization. There would be a fight over the scheme with Hawes on the anti-reform side. Everything depended on Herbert, and Nightingale feared that he was not up to the battle. He was not. In June 1861, he wrote to her that he was dying; by August he was dead. His last words were, "Poor Florence, and our unfinished work."

Nightingale was devastated. She became morose and refused to see anyone. After Herbert's death, progress toward reform took a turn for the worse. Then on November 12, 1861, tragedy struck again. Arthur Clough died. Nightingale mourned in seclusion for a while, but she could not tolerate inaction for long. She went back to work, but now she believed that she worked alone. Her influence in government continued, however.

Lord Palmerston, who had become Prime Minister in 1859, greatly admired her and used his prestige and influence to help her. In May 1862 Hawes died. Nightingale persuaded Palmerston to eliminate Hawes's office of Under Secretary for War and establish in its stead the offices of two under secretaries. These two new offices would be a Military Under Secretary and an Assistant Under Secretary to deal solely with the health administration of the Army. A relative of Nightingale's was appointed to the latter position. In April 1863, the current Secretary for War, George Lewis, died. Nightingale immediately used her influence to obtain the appointment of her longtime friend and supporter, Lord de Gray, as the new Secretary for War. Now at last she was in a position to get things done at the War Office.

Over the next few years the four subcommissions that Nightingale helped create, achieved many reforms. The first subcommission improved construction of new barracks and corrected deficiencies in drainage and ventilation in existing barracks. Water supplies were purified and kitchens were remodeled and sanitized. A School for Practical Cookery was set up to train army cooks to prepare nourishing meals. The second subcommission organized a Statistical Department of the Army that resulted in British Army statistics becoming the best and most complete in Europe. The third subcommission organized an Army Medical School in 1859. Nightingale nominated a number of its professors and contributed to the choice of subjects for the curriculum. The fourth subcommission restructured the Army Medical Department, revised hospital regulations, and drew up a Warrant for the Promotion of Medical Officers. It created regulations for introducing a sanitary code into the army, which was a novel idea for that time. Other Nightingale innovations were the introduction of female nurses into military hospitals and the establishment of soldiers' recreation centers on army posts.

Nightingale's concern for the health of others was not restricted to the Army. In the ten years after the Crimean War, she worked to reform civilian hospitals and workhouse infirmaries in England; to improve health and sanitation in India and other British colonies; and to establish the first professional schools for nurses and midwives. In the years 1856 to 1866 she wrote 45 books and pamphlets concerning sanitation in army and civilian hospitals, hygiene, nursing, statistics, and philosophy. Her 1000-page philosophic treatise, *Suggestions on Thought to Searchers After Truth Among the Artizans of England,* contains her own philosophy, developed from extensive reading of past and current philosophers and from correspondence with some of the outstanding thinkers of her day. In her lifetime she published 147 books and pamphlets concerning sanitation and health. Her personal correspondence was also voluminous.

In 1859, two of Nightingale's best-known books were published, *Notes on Hospitals* and *Notes on Nursing.* These books opened a new era in hospital reforms and health care. In *Notes on Hospitals* she used statistics and inductive reasoning to trace the excessive mortality in hospitals to its true causes: defective sites with improper drainage, overcrowding, and deficient ventilation and light. After the publication of the book her advice was sought and used for hospital construction in England, France, Belgium, Portugal, and India.

Notes on Nursing was written for all women to help them care for their families, but it became a respected text for professional nurses as well. It discussed good hygiene and the prevention of illness as well as care of the sick. In the book she deplored the fact that "...one of every seven infants in...England perished before it was one year old...and two in every five died before they were five years old." She urged mothers to learn the laws of hygiene and use them in rearing their children to prevent illness and death. The principles of nursing she expounded on in this book, such as providing a therapeutic environment for patients, caring for them with empathy, maintaining their confidentiality, and helping them regain their independence as soon as possible, are still basic to nursing.

Until the end of her life Nightingale worked on reforms to improve the health of people. She used statistical data to compile reports explaining the need for each reform that she pursued. She demonstrated how mortality rates increased in institutions with unsanitary conditions. During the process of collecting data on certain hospitals, she recognized a need for uniform statistics on hospitals. Accordingly, she prepared model hospital statistical forms and presented them to the International Statistical Congress in 1860 with a proposal for setting up uniform hospital statistics throughout the world. The Congress approved of her proposal and wrote a resolution that it be communicated to all governments represented there.

Nightingale was still not satisfied. She wanted to help people in their homes as well as in hospitals. She recognized that few people understood the fact that unsanitary conditions in the homes of the poor actually caused disease. She was concerned about the health of people all over the world, not just in England. In 1862 she sent an inquiry to all military stations in India to gather data on the health of the British soldiers living there. The results of the inquiry gave her information on the health of the Indian people as well as on the health of the soldiers. In 1863 she helped write the *Report of the Royal Commission on the Sanitary State of the Army in India.* This two-volume report revealed severe sanitary defects in the living conditions of British soldiers and Indian civilians. In the same year she wrote a report on conditions in other British colonies and published it in a pamphlet, *Sanitary Statistics of Native Colonial Schools and Hospitals.*

Nightingale believed that the problems of people of India and other colonies could only be solved when they were educated to govern themselves. She wrote, "The central idea in dealing with pauperism should be to educate men upwards." In her concern for the people of British colonies, she supported bills for increased self-government and improved local education.

Nightingale's ideas on health and sanitation had far-reaching effects in many areas of social welfare. In the mid-19th century English workhouses were in a sorry state. Crowded together in unsanitary buildings were sick paupers, young children, mentally ill inmates, criminals, and able-bodied paupers. The sick were cared for by the well paupers and the care was of the poorest sort. In January 1864, William Rathbone, a social reformer, wrote to Nightingale to propose a scheme for introducing a team of trained nurses into the Liverpool Workhouse Infirmary. He agreed to pay their salaries if she would select a suitable superintendent. She chose Agnes Jones and sent her with 12 nurses to begin the reform of care of the sick in workhouses.

At the Liverpool Workhouse Jones found unsanitary conditions and overcrowding in the poorly supplied infirmary. Drunkenness was common among the staff, the diet was at starvation level, and linens were often not washed for months. Jones showed the same patience and tact as Nightingale had at Scutari in getting officials to make necessary changes, and the experiment was a success. Nightingale used this success as a lever for promoting larger reforms.

She wrote to the President of the Poor Law Board, describing what had been done in Liverpool and urging him to begin similar systems of nursing in London workhouses. He arranged for Nightingale to work with the Poor Law Inspector for London. She composed a form of inquiry that was issued to all workhouse infirmaries in the city. In 1867 the data she collected was published in her *Suggestions on the Subject of Providing, Training, and Organizing Nurses for the Sick Poor in Workhouse Infirmaries.* In the same year she persuaded the Poor Law Board to pass a Poor Law Reform Bill, which inaugurated reforms in the care of the sick in workhouses. Within ten years all asylums were using paid, trained nurses and the use of pauper nurses eventually became illegal.

In 1867 Nightingale directed her attention to yet another problem. At Kings College Hospital an outbreak of puerperal fever had caused many deaths. She undertook a study of mortality rates of women in childbirth and soon discovered that the death rate in lying-in hospitals was far greater than in private homes. She conducted an inquiry, writing to doctors, matrons, and sanitary engineers all over the world. In 1871, she published *Introductory Notes on Lying-In Institutions,* showing that many lying-in hospitals were poorly run and unsanitary. She advocated isolation of individual patients, sanitary surroundings, and schools for training midwives. This book did for lying-in institutions what *Notes on Hospitals* had done for hospitals in general 12 years before.

Great as these achievements were, Nightingale's greatest contribution to health care reform was her reform of nursing. She recognized a crucial need for educated nurses who would be both committed to serving others and qualified to perform that service. In 1860, through the Nightingale Fund, she established the first professional nursing school at St. Thomas Hospital. It was founded to educate nurses who could act intelligently to prevent illness as well as speed the recovery of patients. At the time the Nightingale Training School was established, Nightingale was a semi-invalid and knew that she could not become an active head of the school. She chose Mrs. Wardroper, whom she greatly admired, to run her school, but she herself masterminded the organization of the school and oversaw the curriculum development.

Before Nightingale reformed nursing, the sick in England were cared for by uneducated personnel. A doctor of the time described nurses as "...dull, unobservant, untaught women; of the best it could only be said that they were kindly and careful and attentive in doing what they were told." Nightingale did not believe that nurses should be dull, unobservant, and just do what they were told. She thought they should be just the opposite—alert, observant, and able to act intelligently and independently. She wrote, "No training is of any use unless one can learn to...think things out for oneself."

Nightingale advocated educating nurses to collect empirical data on patients' conditions through careful observation so that they could make wise judgments about their care. In *Notes on Nursing* she wrote, "The most important practical lesson that can be given to nurses is to teach them what to observe—how to observe—what symptoms indicate improvement—what the reverse—which are of importance—which are of none—which are the evidence of neglect—and of what kind of neglect." She concluded this book by saying, "Pathology teaches the harm that disease has done...nothing more. We know nothing of the principle of health...nothing but observation and experience will teach us the ways to maintain or to bring back the state of health."

Nightingale believed that nursing education should also emphasize the moral development of students. She wrote, "Hospital nursing is the only calling in the world where a woman is really in charge of a number of adults who for purposes of life and death are in their power...Even if you can be sure that a woman has learnt her trade of nurse, you cannot...send her out to such a very responsible situation...till you have trained and tested her as a woman in moral and mental qualities." Nightingale's final assessment of a nurse was that she should be an educated, moral and self-directed individual. She stated, "One must be sure of oneself, of one's character, that it will stand any hour."

Nightingale believed that nursing education should develop both the intellect and the character of the nurse. Accordingly, she gave her students a solid background in the sciences to enable them to understand the theory behind their care. To develop character, she assigned readings in the humanities to increase their understanding of human ethics and morals. She believed that nurses should never stop learning. She wrote to her students, "To nurse is a field of which one may safely say: there is no end in what we may be learning every day."

She envisioned the Nightingale Training School as the germinating source from which a modern profession of nursing would grow. In the first 20 years after the school opened, her graduates became superintendents in many hospitals in Europe, Asia, and the United States. These superintendents often took whole staffs of nurses with them to their new positions, thus introducing a new system of professional nursing.

Nightingale's interest in nursing and health reforms continued to the end of her life. She wrote letters to *The Times* publicizing the need for District Nurses, who could go into the homes of the poor and teach them about hygiene and sanitation. In 1887, in honor of her 50th year of reign, Queen Victoria gave the Women's Jubilee Gift to District Nursing. Nightingale conducted studies and wrote reports on health and sanitation in England until she was well into her 70s, and in her 80s she continued to write letters to her nurses and Crimean War veterans.

Her concern for India also continued into her later years. In the 1870s and 1880s she wrote several articles published in *The Nineteenth Century Magazine,* urging the British government to give the Indian people more representation and freedom to administer their own system of justice and sanitation. In 1889 the Bombay Village Sanitation Act was passed, making each village responsible for educating its citizens. In response to this Act, Nightingale proposed a system of Health Missioners in rural India to educate the people about health and sanitation. This system of missioners was instituted in selected districts of rural India. She helped develop "Village Sanitary Inspection Books" for local officials to use to improve sanitation.

Nightingale was an amazing woman and her accomplishments were prodigious. To better understand her achievements it is necessary to look at her motivations. One needs to examine the ideas that shaped the philosophy behind her sense of mission. She was an avid reader and had an extensive background in history, literature, and philosophy. The writers whose ideas she refers to most in her personal writings are Plato, St. John, Dante, Bacon, Locke, Newton, Kant, Hegel, Comte, and Mill.

Nightingale's philosophy centered on the belief that God had a plan in which everyone was being brought eventually to perfection. She commented, "God's character is to create an eternity in which each one will be on the way through His laws to progress toward perfection." She believed that the world was governed by divinely ordained laws and that people were capable of using their own reason to discern those laws and then use them to improve the condition of the world. She wrote, "God is constantly communicating with us His thought and purpose in law. He gives it not to us except through an appropriate exercise of our faculties. It seems to be the law of God that man should work out the salvation of man."

Nightingale was influenced by the reigning ideas of her time. One of the characteristics of the Victorian era was faith in progress. This idea evolved from discoveries and conclusions of previous periods. Enlightenment thinkers of the 17th century had been so impressed by the ideas and discoveries of men such as

Copernicus, Galileo, Kepler, and Newton that they had come to believe that the human intellect was capable of discovering and using scientific principles to improve human existence. Bacon described the empirical method and Locke popularized it in England, while rationalism developed on the continent. Some 18th-century philosophers were so awed by the power of human reason, they believed that man alone could discover the means of perfecting the world and that there was no further need for divine guidance.

As the 19th century dawned, however, people's glowing confidence in science began to diminish. They saw much in their world that alarmed them and made them recognize a need for ideals as well as material progress. Industrial and political revolutions had brought misery and bloodshed as well as progress. Many Victorians believed that the social order was in grave peril unless people rediscovered and followed higher moral ideals.

In the 19th century a reform spirit grew out of the combination of renewed religious dedication and scientific knowledge. This spirit of reform was given added momentum by idealistic philosophies that filtered into England from Germany. Kant argued that people should be perfected morally as well as materially and that it was God's plan that they should use their reason to work out their perfection. Hegel wrote that the human mind is potential that must be developed by stages until it reaches perfection, and that the perfection of society depends on the ultimate harmony of individual wills with the Universal will. Comte, the father of Positivism in France, advocated using empirical research to discover the social and moral laws to perfect society.

Historians of the 19th century wrote that it was the combined force of scientific knowledge and idealism that enabled reformers of the time to succeed as never before. It was this combination that made Nightingale so successful. She used empirical evidence to illustrate the need for reforms and her belief in philosophic and religious ideals spurred her on to push the needed reforms into reality.

She was influenced by her English heritage, which was steeped in the Empiricist tradition of Bacon and Locke, and by Idealist philosophers who were being popularized in England by her friend Benjamin Jowett, headmaster of Balliol College at Oxford. She agreed with the Idealists and Positivists that God had a plan for people to use their reason to understand the social and moral laws that would lead them to perfection. She felt that it was the duty of enlightened reformers such as herself to help people understand those laws so that God's plan could be fulfilled. She greatly admired Hegel and Comte and commented on them in a letter to her father, "Hegel and Comte are men who...have a grasp of absolute truth never before equaled."

Nightingale's beliefs were also shaped by Unitarian ideas. She was brought up in a Unitarian family, and her own writings show the influence of Unitarian concepts. She agreed with the Unitarians that religion should concern itself with action for the benefit of others. She wrote, "Organize your life to act out your religion." Unitarians believed that God had given all people the wisdom to work out their own perfection either in this life or the life to come. They emphasized the importance of education in developing each person's divine potential. Nightingale agreed with their belief that education was vital for preparing people to understand God's laws for the perfection of mankind.

Three contemporary intellectuals, John Stuart Mill, Benjamin Jowett, and Harriet Martineau, also had strong influences on Nightingale's ideas. Mill critiqued her philosophic book, *Suggestions for Thought.* She told Mill that his book, *A System of Logic,* was the forming influence on both her book and herself. She agreed with Mill that people could learn social laws from the experiences of others in history and could use these laws to accelerate human progress. She was a student of history and felt that knowledge of failures of past civilizations could help people improve their own societies. Nightingale, like Hegel and Mill, believed that the study of history could lead people to greater and greater insights into the ultimate truths of the Universal Mind. Once people knew and followed these truths, the perfection of society would follow.

Jowett shared an interest in philosophy with Nightingale. They wrote letters over a 30-year period discussing the philosophies of Plato and Hegel at length, as well as education, politics, and religion. Jowett's biographer, Geoffrey Faber, describes him as fascinated by Nightingale because of her possession of an intellect equal to and not dissimilar from his own. From his deathbed he wrote to her, "How large a part has your life been of my life." She replied, "It does make a great difference to my life to know that you are in the world...You do do me good."

Martineau wrote editorials for the *Daily News* and had a number of books published, including her translation of Comte's *The Positive Philosophy.* She and Nightingale discussed people, philosophy, women's issues, politics, and other issues in their correspondence.

The people in Nightingale's family who had the most positive influence on her ideas were her father and her Aunt Mai. Both of them were interested in speculative philosophy and conversed at length with her about philosophic ideas. Mr. Nightingale was well educated and, like other Unitarians, held views about the importance of educating women, which were much in advance of the common opinion of the time. He gave Nightingale an extensive liberal education. She learned several languages and read widely in ancient and modern history and philosophy. She was also a serious student of the Bible. When she was entering adulthood she went on vacations with her family and friends to Europe and Egypt. During their travels she was introduced to some of the outstanding intellectuals of the time and she later corresponded with a number of them.

Florence's Aunt Mai was especially fond of her and understood her need to apply her intelligence and drive in worthwhile pursuits. They discussed their philosophic ideas in letters and in person. Aunt Mai left her own family for a while to support her niece when she was ill and desperately needed to finish her work on reforming the health administration of the Army.

Other family members had a less positive influence on Florence's life. She believed that her mother and her sister, Parthe, were hindrances to the achievement of her life's goals. When she felt called by God to do hospital work, they fought her doing this for many years because they thought that nursing was below her social status. The first third of Florence's life was a series of anguished conflicts between them and herself as she tried to break the bond of filial duty imposed on her by their Victorian attitudes.

The long struggle to break loose from her family left Florence bitter about the Victorian view of women. The intensity of her feeling poured out in her writings. In one of her books she questioned the manner in which parents in her society treated their daughters. She wrote, "Did they bring them into the world to be their bounden slaves as long as they live, unless they can be gratified by a marriage to their taste?" After the Crimean War she wrote a stinging criticism of the treatment she had received from her sister.

Her mother's and sister's influences on her were not, perhaps, entirely negative. Their resistance to her pursuit of her goals may have strengthened her determination to become a nurse and given her the perseverance she needed to accomplish reforms. She was able to surmount the enervating effect of her environment and to resolve the depression it had induced by dedicating herself to an ideal, a life of service.

The most important element in Nightingale's success was her personality. She was influenced by the popular concepts of her time and by close personal associations, but the uniqueness of her personality determined the manner in which she responded to others and the world around her. Some of her most distinctive traits were her perfectionism, her brilliance, and her drive. She was intense, determined, and an able administrator. Her religious faith gave her strength of conviction and singleness of purpose.

Nightingale's perfectionist nature was a lifelong stimulus. She never felt that she was deserving enough to please God, so she strove continually to perfect herself in His eyes. She wrote to

Jowett, "I think if I could have felt God loved me, I could have born anything. But I never could feel it." Her repeated plea in private notes was, "Oh God, conduct me now—do Thou bring good out of this failure."

Nightingale believed that people could only move toward perfection by letting God's will take over their hearts and minds. She prayed, "Lord, we would have no will but Thine and we would try actively to do Thy will, and be about our Father's business always." She felt that she was a coworker with God carrying out His mission to perfect mankind. When she was 52, she wrote, "O my Creator...Thou knowest that through all these twenty years I have been supported and only supported by the belief that I was working with Thee who wert bringing everyone to perfection."

Another key factor in Nightingale's success was her brilliance. She had a remarkable ability to grasp the essentials of large amounts of statistical data and clearly present her findings. Her Aunt Mai commented, "You cannot think of what it is to watch a great mind like hers at work and fully equal to that great work." Queen Victoria was impressed with her powerful mind and sought her advice on many issues.

Intellectual pursuits were not enough to satisfy Nightingale, however. She had a drive for action and wanted a productive part in working out God's plan for mankind. This drive to carry out ideals in action spurred Nightingale on to be one of the greatest reformers of the 19th century. Nightingale's brilliance and drive won the support of progressive thinkers and helped her persevere when there was resistance to needed reforms.

Nightingale also had some negative personality traits. She was extremely demanding of others and often lost sight of their personal needs. She was impatient with anyone who got in the way of her mission, especially her mother and sister. Her impatience with them left her with feelings of guilt, which were not assuaged until after she nursed them through long illnesses at the ends of their lives.

Another interesting aspect of Nightingale's personality was her unwillingness to marry and raise a family. She denied herself family life to devote her life to a larger cause. In her 20s she turned down two proposals of marriage from eligible suitors, Henry Nicolson and Richard Moncton Milnes. She believed that "...few marriages were perfect and that generally marriage meant the sacrifice of higher qualities in a woman to the satisfaction of the lower qualities." Concerning the raising of children, she commented, "To me, the idea of modifying children's natures has always appeared too immeasurably awful to perform." She was not afraid to tackle the task of reforming mankind, but she was wary of trying to shape the individual lives of her own children.

Nightingale never held an official position in the government, yet she was able to bring about far-reaching reforms in the administration of her government and other governments for the betterment of society. She believed that everyone should be helped through education to develop his or her potential. She wanted this for soldiers, civilians, and nurses, rich or poor. Perhaps her mission was impossible to achieve, but in striving toward it she improved the human condition of her world.

Unless otherwise noted, all quotations are from manuscripts in the Nightingale collection in the Manuscript Room of the British Library in London.

REFLECTIONS ON NIGHTINGALE'S PERSPECTIVE OF NURSING.

Joyce J. Fitzpatrick

To say that we are indebted to Nightingale for her vision of nursing is an understatement because Nightingale can be credited with planting the seeds that blossomed into the current understanding of nursing as both science and art. The following statements reflect my analysis of Nightingale's contributions, with particular attention to the congruence of Nightingale's vision with the life-perspective–rhythm paradigm of people, their environments, and their health. In particular, the relevance of Nightingale's laws of health, her holistic view of people, and the posited relationships between environmental factors and health are examined in relation to the key concepts within the rhythm model. Finally, Nightingale's principles relevant to both the process and the content of development of ways of knowing in nursing are addressed.

Even before I began a thorough study of the philosophic and theoretical dimensions of Nightingale's work, I was impressed, and in fact awed, by her contributions to nursing. Nightingale is inspiring, on first glance and every glance thereafter. As a person Nightingale challenged the status quo; as a leader in health care reform Nightingale used her influence and power to change the system. As an advocate for the sick and the well Nightingale spread the word to hundreds of women that to care for others, to minister to the ill, and to teach the principles of disease prevention and wellness was a special calling, a vocation that was to be followed. I was impressed most of all with her persistence, her

Joyce J. Fitzpatrick, Ph.D., R.N., F.A.A.N., is Professor and Dean of Nursing at the Frances Payne Bolton School of Nursing, Case Western Reserve University, Cleveland, Ohio.

tenacity in the midst of social pressures and considerable obstacles to achievement of her goals. Nightingale's commitment to her own ideals led to her success; she was driven beyond the reasonable and not easily discouraged by the day-to-day frustrations that might have stopped a weaker soul.

NIGHTINGALE'S LAWS OF HEALTH.

Nightingale's observational skills were well developed and she encouraged the refinement of observational skills among the nurses she trained, whether they were to care for the sick or to teach wellness. As a result of her attention to observation, Nightingale's laws of health are grounded in the observables, and often tied to environmental factors such as dampness and dirt. Nightingale's science and clinical practice are thus rooted in empiricism, which continues to be the predominant scientific methodology used today. This prevailing value for empiricism is entirely consistent with the view that I have held of scientific development within nursing, that is, that we should fully embrace the predominant scientific view within our culture, at the same time forging new discoveries through experimentation with cutting-edge methods. Nightingale's science was epidemiologic in nature; she used her understandings of disease pathology in combination with a thorough knowledge of statistics to describe the morbidity and mortality in regional areas. This global perspective on illness gave her a deeper understanding of the factors that influence health and illness, and helped to structure her understanding of the significant factors altering an individual patient's health.

Nightingale's laws of health include health as both the absence of disease and the use of personal power; thus, health can be understood as more than the opposite of disease and within the broader wellness paradigm. Certainly the emphasis for Nightingale is on the aspect of health as related to illness, but her openness to the power component of health is particularly consistent with a life-perspective model of human health and development. Within this paradigm, the proposed relationship is that people derive meaning from life experiences and the extent to which life has meaning influences the person's health status. For Nightingale health could be augmented through education. To the extent that the education consists of personal insights and personal growth and development, this view is consistent with my proposed views on health. Furthermore, Nightingale viewed disease as a reparative process, an effort on the part of the body to seek some harmony and to gain some spiritual perspective. To a large extent this Nightingale view is consistent with the life-perspective–rhythm model.

NIGHTINGALE'S HOLISTIC VIEW OF PEOPLE.

Nightingale viewed people holistically even though her attention to the physical aspects of health and illness was most predominant. Second to the physical dimension, Nightingale placed emphasis on the spiritual dimension. She viewed a person as including physical, intellectual, emotional, social, and spiritual components. Furthermore, Nightingale viewed people as equal, regardless of birth right, social class, or biologic differences. She truly believed in the dignity and sanctity of human life. Nightingale's view of the value of human life is most consistent with the beliefs and attitudes that predominate within professional nursing today. She selected the philosophic path that we continue to travel and designed the overall structure for the profession of nursing. Her core values remain with us today.

For Nightingale, the holistic nature of people was more of an additive or complementary approach, in contrast to the view of holism as "greater than the sum of the parts." One of the most striking aspects of Nightingale's view of people is her attitude of caring for the person who is ill rather than being concerned about the illness per se. This attitude reflects the distinguishing aspect of professional nursing. In this regard Nightingale reflected the essence of professional nursing practice, emphasizing the unique interpersonal relationship that the nurse has with his or her patient to influence health. Although Nightingale does not detail the components of the relationship itself, she implies that it is highly individualized, intense, helpful to the patient, and satisfying to the nurse.

RELATIONSHIPS BETWEEN ENVIRONMENTAL FACTORS AND HEALTH.

To Nightingale environment is central. It serves as a key factor in preventing diseases and in restoring health when disease has occurred. Many of Nightingale's instructions to nurses included information about environmental manipulations to influence the health and comfort of the patient. Her posited laws of nature described ways in which the environment could affect the patient's health. She placed a special emphasis on five elements of the environment in relation to health; these included cleanliness, light, pure air, pure water, and efficient drainage.

In her view of environment, Nightingale was able to express the relationship among the health and person concepts: a person's health (or illness) was a result of the environmental influences on him or her. The environment was the encompassing context in which people lived. Nightingale's view of environment reflected a dual system perspective rather than a perspective that treated person and environment as consistent aspects of one system. In an open system perspective of people, environment becomes a less central concept because it is indistinguishable form the core person concept. Person becomes the central concept, and it is as if the environment is an essential characteristic of the person. In contrast to the life-perspective–rhythm model, which telescopes the individual for intensive conceptual development, Nightingale telescoped the larger perspective. She extended her focus on the environment during her extensive analysis of the sanitary conditions during the Crimean War and the sanitary conditions of hospitals in general. She was concerned about not only the negative environmental conditions in hospitals but also the organization, construction, and management of hospitals. Thus, her view of environment was broad. Furthermore, Nightingale was consistent throughout her writings in her emphasis on the environmental influences on health. She set the stage for the later attention to public health nursing and the more contemporary focus on public health policy.

PROCESS AND CONTENT OF KNOWING IN NURSING.

Most impressive and instructive to me in my repeated analysis of Nightingale's influence on nursing today is the scope of her influence and the extent to which her teachings appear timeless. Also significant is Nightingale's integration of elements of both science and clinical practice in her understanding of what it is important for nurses to know. Nightingale believed it is critical for the nurse to be knowledgeable about factors influencing health and illness and to be totally committed to her patients; for Nightingale nursing is a calling, a vocation. Thus, Nightingale expected that nurses would know in multiple ways: by applying scientific principles, by observing the laws of nature, and by caring for the patients who required assistance in restoring their health. Nursing education represented an alternative for women, to prepare them for new ways of knowing and new ways of caring.

Nightingale's perspective on nursing continues to represent a challenging view of the potential for changing our understanding of the health and human experiences. Her emphasis on the development of science about health and illness has served as a constant reminder to me of our strivings to know more about the human experience, especially those conditions that lead to disease and death. Although her science has been instructive, by far the most significant aspects of her teaching for me have been the personal and professional qualities she so aptly demonstrated in her work and in her writing. Nightingale has been an inspiration to countless nurses as they continue to ask the deeper questions that push the scientific doors open a little more, and more importantly, as they instill the spirit of clinical inquiry and the passionate zeal for making the lives of others better through nursing care. I am only one of millions of nurses who have benefited from her leadership and vision.

THE ORIGINS OF THE BEHAVIORAL SYSTEM MODEL.

Dorothy E. Johnson

Notes on Nursing came into my life early in my teaching experience when the publisher's representative gave me a copy of the facsimile edition published in 1946. It came just at the right time to have a profound influence on the course of my professional experience. I had just begun to develop the clinical courses in a baccalaureate program for which I was newly responsible, and I was struggling to identify the content appropriate for those courses and how it should be organized. I had course outlines for the courses as they had been previously taught and I had completed very similar courses in my own preparation. It was also evident in a general way what was expected of a practicing nurse in the clinical area. These pragmatic approaches to selecting content seemed to me to be most unsatisfactory, however.

The course content previously offered was what seemed to me to be medical science; it consisted of a lengthy exposition of the etiology, pathology, and treatment of a particular disease or group of diseases, usually taught by a physician, followed by a shorter presentation of the implications of the disease and its treatment for nursing care. Nursing care as presented in the classroom and as seen in the hospital setting, was dictated for the most part by the physician's orders or hospital procedures and routines. Of course, in my own preparation as well as in the current teaching situation, instructors were careful to also draw attention to the psychological and social needs of patients and their families, but these discussions, presumably based on the

Dorothy E. Johnson, R.N., M.P.H., is Professor Emerita from the School of Nursing, University of California, Los Angeles, California.

social sciences, often seemed to be simply exhortations of a general nature, such as the importance of relieving anxiety.

My own educational experience had led me to believe that nursing was a profession, or at least an emerging one, and that as a profession nursing makes a unique and significant contribution to patients—a contribution that differs from but is complementary to those made by medicine and other health professions. We also learned the other major attributes of a profession, including the responsibility for the continuous development of the scientific bases for practice, and we were encouraged to find ways to contribute to the expansion of nursing knowledge. It seemed evident to me, as a young teacher, that based on this understanding of the profession of nursing, the content in nursing courses should derive from the profession's unique contribution to patient welfare, not from medicine's contribution or the routines and procedures established by hospitals. Unfortunately I could find no clear, concise answer to the question of nursing's explicit goal in patient care, at least not one on which there seemed to be widespread agreement. If nursing is not exactly what nurses are taught, or what nurses do, then what is it?

Florence Nightingale, writing in *Notes on Nursing,* provided direction to my thinking. She did not emphasize knowledge of disease, although she did not say it was unimportant. She did not emphasize hospital routines or procedures, or at least not in their own right. Rather she stated quite clearly that the word nursing "...ought to signify the proper use of fresh air, light, warmth, cleanliness, quiet, and the proper selection and administration of diet—all at the least expense of vital power to the patient" (p. 6). She goes further to lament that "...those laws which God has assigned to the relations of our bodies with the world in which he has put them" (p. 7) were only partially known, but to the extent known, were "...all but unlearnt" (p. 7). These two points—a focus on the basic human needs of the person and a concern for the relationship between the person and the environment—provided the beginning of the development of the behavioral system framework for nursing.

Over the next 20 years the development of this framework went through a number of stages as it evolved. The work began with the effort to develop course content in the basic curriculum by focusing on common human needs, moving on to "care and comfort" as organizing principles, and then to stress and tension reduction as the major principles. These developments were reported in conferences and through the literature as they took place through the 1950s. The focus on the person and his or her needs per se was not completely satisfactory for a number of reasons, most notably the difficulty in specifying the patient outcomes that result from nursing's service. Moreover, the emphasis seemed to be wrongly placed on the patient as a passive recipient of services rather than as an active and reactive participant in his or her own care.

It was Nightingale's emphasis on the relationship of the person to his or her environment that led to a consideration of a system approach as a scientifically viable and professionally sound means of resolving these difficulties. Medicine had been using a biologic system approach in patient care for some time with considerable success both scientifically and in practice. Sociologists and social workers were discussing social systems. Why not, for nursing's purposes, behavioral systems? The emphasis on basic human needs need not and should not be discarded, but human needs could be viewed from a different, more useful perspective. Each of the needs Nightingale specified could be seen as a way of interacting with the environment, and the interdependence between the needs and between the needs and the environment could be easily conceptualized.

It was perhaps not exactly fortuitous, but it was certainly important that at this stage in my thinking, in the late 1950s and early 1960s, an increasing number of observational studies of behavioral patterns of children and adults as well as animal groups were appearing in the literature. These reports from child developmentalists, sociologists, psychologists, anthropologists, and animal behaviorists varied in the way the behavioral patterns were organized and classified, but there was a certain commonality in the behaviors selected for observation. Simultaneously a heightened awareness of the possibility of general system theory was appearing in the literature; these papers were coming from social as well as physical and biologic scientists. Although general system theory was in its infancy, it did seem valid enough to support the notion of humans as behavioral systems, developing and changing, reacting and adapting to their respective environments, including other behavioral systems in that environment. It also became possible to conceptualize nursing's unique contribution as that of protecting, supporting, and fostering necessary and desired change in the behavioral systems of the people we serve.

By beginning with the fundamental needs of people identified by Nightingale as significant, and enriching and changing these as the literature seemed to indicate, the picture of the behavioral system and its subsystems gradually began to emerge. All the patterned, repetitive, purposeful ways of behaving that characterize each person's life were conceptualized as forming an organized and integrated whole—a system. This system determines and limits the interaction between the person and his or her environment and establishes the relationship of the person to the objects, events, and situations in the environment. The behavioral system has many tasks or missions to perform in maintaining its own integrity and in managing the system's relationship to the environment; thus, the parts of the system evolve or subsystems develop, each to perform its specialized tasks for the system as a whole.

Each subsystem is formed by a set of behavioral responses, or responsive tendencies, or action systems, that seem to share a common drive or goal. Organized around drives (or some type of intraorganismic motivational structure), these responses are differentiated, developed, and modified over time through maturation, experiences, and learning. They are determined and continuously governed by a multitude of physical, biologic, psychological, and social factors operating in a complex and interlocking fashion. The subsystems now identified are those that seem to be of major adaptive significance; they are attachment or affiliative behavior, dependency behavior, ingestive behavior, eliminative behavior, aggressive behavior, sexual behavior, and achievement behavior.

Admittedly even now knowledge about the behavioral patterns in the response or action systems is greater than knowledge of the underlying structures, and knowledge about the parts or subsystems is greater than knowledge of the system as a whole. Nonetheless, the body of knowledge about the behavioral system and its subsystems is sufficiently substantial to allow pertinent observations and useful interpretations in practice. It also points to many possibilities for intervention as well as avenues for research. In this way a body of knowledge about disorders in the behavioral system and their prevention and treatment will be developed and expanded over time and will be known as nursing science.

It was in regard to prevention that Nightingale's thinking further illuminated my own work. She equated what she called the laws of health with the laws of nursing. I could not agree with her on this point, since both my basic preparation in public health nursing and my graduate work in public health persuaded me that nurses share with all members of the health team a general responsibility for the health of society, with preventive medicine, sanitary engineering, health education, and the like each playing its part. Nightingale's emphasis on health *and* nursing forced me to clarify my thinking about nursing's special contribution to the health of society. In time I began to recognize that nursing's special responsibility for health is derived from its unique social mission. Although nursing and nurses would always contribute to the health of society by using, when appropriate, the knowledge and skills of other health team members, nursing would need to concentrate on developing preventive nursing to fulfill its social obligations.

With the behavioral system orientation nursing would have a special responsibility to promote the most effective and efficient behavioral system possible, as well as to prevent specific problems from occurring in the system. Meeting this responsibility would also contribute to healthier biologic and social systems. Clarifying nursing's social mission through an explicit goal in patient care and using a specific body of knowledge relevant to that goal therefore enables the discipline to work toward completing its special tasks in prevention, thus contributing to a high level of wellness in society.

One additional comment is in order. The content of *Notes on Nursing* is drawn not only from Nightingale's personal experiences in nursing, but also from her significant studies of morbidity and mortality rates and her observations of sanitary conditions and their possible relationship to disease. She was truly nursing's first scholar. Although many of the comments she makes here have been shown to be in error, it is most often in the conclusions reached rather than the observations themselves. Her chapter entitled "Variety," for example, was surely the forerunner of all the scientific work on sensory deprivation, sensory monotony, and sensory overload. The chief contributions to nursing made by this little book, however, were Nightingale's focus on the person rather than the disease and her emphasis on the significance of the environment for the person's well-being. She clearly saw nursing's social mission as different from that of medicine, and nursing's role as one of personal service to people.

In the face of the many distractions and potential obstacles nurses face in meeting their individual and group responsibilities to fulfill the legacy Nightingale left, it is wise to be reminded of these responsibilities periodically by rereading *Notes on Nursing*. Clearly I feel personally indebted to Nightingale for the concepts of nursing she offered. More importantly, however, the profession might have evolved in a very different way or even disappeared, at least under the name nursing, without Nightingale's timely leadership and scholarship.

REFLECTIONS ON NIGHTINGALE WITH A FOCUS ON HUMAN CARE THEORY AND LEADERSHIP.

Madeleine Leininger

Let us always be open to acknowledge, respect, and learn from great leaders in any field or discipline. Let us always be able to critique the work of any leader to move forward ideas and substantive knowledge for the betterment of humanity. For, indeed, great progress is largely contingent upon thoughtful reflections, critiques, and the creative use of worthwhile ideas.

It was this philosophic statement that led me to reflect on Florence Nightingale's contributions to human care as expressed in her well-known book, *Notes on Nursing*. This small but thought-provoking book, written in 19th century prose, has lead many nurses to read and reflect on her ideas over the past hundred years. It reflects Victorian British cultural norms, values, and the environmental context in which Nightingale lived most of her life.

WHAT NIGHTINGALE SAID OR FAILED TO SAY ABOUT CARE/CARING.

Although the book shows that Nightingale made a number of noteworthy and pioneering contributions that lay the foundations for professional nursing education and practice, there con-

---

Madeleine Leininger, R.N., C.T.N., Ph.D., L.H.D., D.S., Ph.DNsc., F.A.A.N. is Professor of Nursing and Anthropology in the Colleges of Nursing and Liberal Arts, Wayne State University, Detroit, Michigan.

tinue to be a number of outstanding nurse leaders who have made comparable contributions in each unfolding era in nursing. Nightingale was, however, the brave, bold, and great risk-taking leader who served as a model of how to make breakthroughs in nursing and establish new standards, directions, and practices. Every true leader faces similar challenges to carve new pathways to nursing knowledge and practice. Indeed, some leaders claim that each decade it gets more difficult because of the many complex and diverse cultural forces that have to be dealt with in any institution, society, or worldwide system. Overcoming such challenges or obstacles is the sign of a true leader, however.

As one of many leaders in nursing, I have been faced with many challenges in developing and establishing the transcultural nursing field with human care as the central focus. In addition, I developed and refined qualitative methods to document the epistemics and ontologic realities of nursing when there were virtually no supporters or workers interested in this approach. I can attest to the fact that leadership must not only be creative but also persistent and have a deep commitment and vision for what might be best for nursing, society, and humanity. The opportunity to travel and to learn about many different kinds of "Nightingales" and other leaders in the United States, Africa, South American, Europe, Southeast Asia, Oceania, and other places around the world gave me a deep appreciation for outstanding leaders, many of whom are still largely unknown in the nursing world. These limitedly recognized nurses are making some distinctive leadership contributions that could well surpass Nightingale's to advance the discipline and profession of nursing.

In this paper, I will briefly assess Nightingale's perspectives about human care and then contrast them with my theory of Culture Care and ongoing contributions related to care over the past four decades. I will compare and contrast the leadership attributes of Nightingale and myself.

Today human care has at last become the central focus of nursing knowledge and practice, grounded in the explication of embedded meanings, patterns, and interpretations from both client and nurse perspectives.

Moreover, many professional nurses have liberated themselves from a heavy focus on medical symptoms, diseases, and treatment modes to focusing on discovering and understanding the nature, meanings, and life experiences related to human caring. The tremendous importance and power of care to heal, restore, and maintain well-being is being realized by care scholars. The shift to a focus on human care and caring has occurred mainly in recent decades because of a cadre of committed nurse scholars, theoreticians, clinicians, and researchers who have sought to study care in a systematic and rigorous way since the mid-1950s (Aamodt, 1978; Gaut, 1981; Leininger, 1970; 1977;

1978; 1981; 1984; 1988; 1991; Watson, 1979; 1985). As a central leader who has spearheaded this cultural care movement and committed most of my professional and academic career to research and teaching of human care, I can attest to the growing excitement today as new and seasoned nurses discover the significance of human caring in health and well-being.

It was in the 1950s that I began to proclaim, "Care is the essence of nursing and the dominant, and unifying domain of nursing" (Leininger, 1970; 1977; 1981). Since then, I have been frequently confronted about Nightingale's views on humanistic and scientific care in relation to my theory and research. Nursing students often ask, "What really were Nightingale's views about human care? What evidence is there that Nightingale valued and practiced care in *Notes on Nursing*? Can care be inferred from Nightingale's statements and prescriptions of how a nurse should or ought to function? In what ways did cultural values and gender influence Nightingale's thinking about nursing practices?" These questions and others led to my reexamination of Nightingale's classic book of 1859.

Interestingly, Nightingale never defined human care or caring in *Notes on Nursing,* but she made inferences about treating the sick in the hospital environment. She made many proscriptions and rules for nurses about what to do for sick patients. Clearly, Nightingale's recurrent concepts in *Notes on Nursing* were *health, hygiene,* and *environment.* She never defined nor gave interpretations of these key terms, however, but spoke about health principles and "laws of health" as imperatives for the nurse (pp. 14, 73, 75). She identified the five essential points to secure health: pure air, pure water, efficient drainage, cleanliness, and light (p. 14). These areas are emphasized throughout the book, particularly cleanliness, fresh air (sunlight), food, and a clean environment to restore patients to health. She stated, "...what constitutes good nursing are little understood for the well as for the sick. The same laws of health or of nursing, for they are in reality the same, obtain among the well as among the sick" (p. 6). Health was viewed as the same as nursing, and care was not discussed in relation to health.

Nightingale's philosophy of nursing and action modality was "to put the patient in the best condition for nature to act upon him" (p. 75). This statement was profound for the times, because it clearly identified both a new way to help the sick and the central role of the nurse to place patients in an environment where nature could restore them back to health. Nature was a curing, restorative force and the nurse provided or monitored the environment with a clean and quiet setting, proper food, and limited noise and offensive odors. The five essential factors and Nightingale's philosophy of health were the *sine qua non* for nursing practice.

According to Nightingale, the nurse's role was also to make "habitual" observations and recordings and to monitor the sick patient's condition in the environment to support *nature* to act on the restorative processes (p. 6). She helped nurses see that the incidents of a disease were usually not the symptoms of the disease but something quite different, namely, the need for fresh air, light, warmth, diet, or cleanliness of the patient (p. 5). Whether nursing care decisions and actions figured into the reparative process with nature as the powerful means was never explicitly stated. One wonders if Nightingale considered components of care such as comfort, support, nurturance, and many other care constructs and characteristics and how they would influence the reparative process. Were nature and the five health essentials more important than the use of care constructs? Nightingale did not clarify these ideas.

Using my theory of Culture Care Diversity and Universality, many care constructs have been discovered from both the client's and nurse's meanings and uses. Great diversity exists in care constructs with 54 cultures and with the meanings and practices of care (Gaut, 1981; Leininger, 1981; 1984; 1988; 1991; Luna, 1989; Stasiak, 1991; Wenger, 1991). For the first time in the history of nursing implicit and explicit cultural care meanings, forms, patterns, and expressions of care have been documented and valued for their impact on the health and the well-being of clients. The expressions and meanings of care and caring were largely embedded in the client's world view, social structure, ethnohistory, linguistic expressions, and environmental context. Of great interest is that the nurse used the terms "care," "caring," and "nursing care" like cliches or magical terms in nursing without fully knowing their meanings to himself or herself or to clients. Transcultural nurse researchers have been able to identify some of the culture-specific meanings, forms, and practices related to generic and professional care (Leininger, 1981; 1988; 1991). These care constructs are being used in specific ways to guide professional nursing decisions and actions to provide culturally congruent care. In addition, *care-giving* and *care-receiving* knowledge among the client, his or her nurse, and family members is being used to improve nursing care practices. Such care research findings are providing a whole new body of knowledge to guide nursing practices since Nightingale's *Notes on Nursing*. The theory of Culture Care, along with transcultural nursing principles and concepts, has been important in the shift of nursing into caring science and the transformation of nursing education and practice.

As one looks further at Nightingale's ideas about care, one can identify several inferences about care, especially with respect to the nurse's role.

> *All hurry or bustle is peculiarly painful to the sick...Always sit down when a sick person is talking business to you, show no signs of hurry, give complete attention and full consideration if your advice is wanted...Always sit within the patient's view, so that when you speak to him he has not painfully to turn his head round in order to look at you...Never speak to an invalid from behind, nor from the door, nor from any distance...(p. 28).*

These statements could be interpreted as *giving presence and attention to* the client as a caring modality.

Nightingale gave other directives, rules, and proscriptions that could be questioned today, however. They include beneficial caring modalities such as "Conciseness and decision are, above all things, necessary with the sick," and "Let your doubt be to yourself, your decision to them" (p. 31). These rules reflect the cultural norms of Nightingale's day—to be directive, firmly in control of a situation, and authoritative in decision making. Many clients in American culture today would not like this approach; they expect nurses to respect their ideas and decisions. A nurse with a caring attitude and knowledge must understand the client's perspectives and wishes and function in a coparticipant way rather than take an authoritative stance. Care decisions for many clients are made *with* rather than *for* the client. Moreover, nurses using care principles and insights will often wait for the client and his or her family to make decisions so that care fits with or is reasonably congruent with the client's culture, values, beliefs, and lifeways. Nursing as a caring process is to discover *with* the client diverse factors and environmental resources to help the client regain and maintain well-being. Noncaring behaviors, attitudes, and practices are often identified by clients in United States hospitals when they fail to understand generic or local care expectations.

Throughout *Notes on Nursing* Nightingale stated proscriptions for the nurse's responsibilities to the sick patient with an emphasis on the nurse making the environment proper for the patient. Among these directives were a host of things to attend to in order to "spare" the patient even in "taking thought for himself" (p. 63). The hospital as the environment was to be managed to relieve the patient "from all anxiety, afforded by the rules of a well-regulated institution, which has often such a beneficial effect upon the patient" (p. 63). There were many examples of what a "good" nurse was to *do for the patient* for the reparative process to occur in the hospital environment. Interestingly, *self-care* was not the order or proscription of the Nightingale era. Instead, the nurse was to *do things for the patients* since the nurse was expected to know what was best for them. Again, these values reflected the British Victorian culture of the 19th century.

Using my Culture Care theory, I have documented that many non-Western clients seek and want nurses to support *other care* in which family members are active partners in care (Leininger, 1988; 1991). But today, American nurses are fostering *self-care* practices to meet self-care deficits that may not always be congruent with client needs and expectations (Orem, 1980). Transcultural nurse researchers have also identified the importance of family members as generic caregivers that contrast with professional care practices. These latter ideas of generic and professional care were never identified in Nightingale's work but today are clearly important in professional nursing education and practice.

Looking further at Nightingale's ideas about care patterns and ideas in the 19th century, one finds that she saw patients as passive, shy, and dependent on the nurse, and believed that sick patients needed to be acted on and receive help from the nurse. She also felt that it was unwise for patients to focus on *their condition*. She stated:

I cannot too often repeat that patients are generally either too languid to observe these things (reference to food and other physical needs), or too shy to speak about them; nor is it well that they should be made to observe them, it fixes their attention upon themselves (p. 62).

Nightingale seemed quite concerned about sick patients dwelling on their condition, which she believed would limit their restorative processes. Although this was an important psychological care consideration, it contrasts sharply with many middle and upper class Anglo-American clients or with clients from other cultures, who often demand, expect, or want to know explicitly their health conditions, treatment modes, and what might happen to them. Nurses are, therefore, expected to be well-informed about the client and knowledgeable about his or her condition, and to share any new developments that could influence the client's health or perceived well-being state.

Throughout the book, Nightingale gives her cultural beliefs—norms, desired standards, prescribed roles, and functions to help the sick patient. She repeatedly emphasizes the responsibility of the nurse to make detailed and continuous recorded observations of the sick in their environment while at the same time provide practical and common-sense ways to support the patient's reparative healing process. Surveillance and direct observations remain extremely important *caring* characteristics of a caring nurse. Among Nightingale's admonitions and directives was her emphasis on the need for nurses to make habitual observations:

For it may safely be said, not that the habit of ready and correct ob-
servation will by itself make us useful nurses, but that without it
we shall be useless with all our devotion...but if you cannot get the
habit of observation one way or other, you had better give up the be-
ing a nurse, for it is not your calling, however kind and anxious
you may be (p. 63).

This was a strong mandate for being a nurse, and Nightingale linked it to the nurse's unique role responsibilities and functions of observing, attending to, and providing direct and
continuous services to the sick in their environment. The caring
modalities related to surveillance, watchfulness, safety, attention to, concern for (or about), and presence can be inferred as
crucial to being a good nurse.

Most encouragingly, Nightingale stressed that nurses had
role responsibilities that were *distinct from those of medicine.*
This statement was of great importance to advance not only the
discipline and profession of nursing but to provide the context for
caring to occur. Today there are nurses in many places in the
world who continue to imitate physicians and medical practices
and fail to see nursing as a profession in its own right, with its
own body of knowledge. This knowledge to characterize and le-
gitimize nursing as a discipline is human *care*, which, I have
theorized, leads to *health* and *well-being* in different cultural and
environmental contexts. Nurses need to practice care to be
nurses, and nursing requires some autonomous decisions and actions that are different from physicians, who focus on medical
diseases, symptoms, and curing. Nightingale indeed was a wise
and perceptive leader who envisioned nursing becoming a distinct field from medicine. This distinction was important in establishing caring science knowledge to guide nursing actions and
decisions. Nightingale used her "concise and precise" decisions as
means to exert her authority and control over nursing practices
and to hold her own with physicians. She used detailed recordings and observations as well as instructions to the physician as
a means to control nursing practices.

As I considered my theory of Culture Care, it appeared interesting to me that while Nightingale provided heroic nursing
services to the men wounded in the Crimean War, she neither
discussed nor considered culture care factors related to nursing.
Occasionally she spoke of sick patients who were "peculiar" but
without recognizing cultural differences or similarities. She also
did some traveling but limitedly drew on cultural experiences in
nursing education and practice. Thus, the body of culture-specific
care knowledge and practice is a significant development since
Nightingale's time.

A COMPARISON OF LEININGER'S CULTURAL CARE THEORY WITH NIGHTINGALE'S BELIEFS.

A complete discussion of my theory of Culture Care has been presented in a recent publication with the ethnonursing research method and research findings (Leininger, 1991); therefore, only highlights are discussed here and contrasted with Nightingale's beliefs.

The theory of Culture Care differs considerably from Nightingale's in that I have focused on the systematic and in-depth study of culture care values, beliefs, meanings, and practices with respect to differences and similarities among diverse cultures in the world. The purpose of the theory is to describe, explain, and interpret *emic* (local or internal) and *etic* (external) human care phenomena as known and experienced by designated cultures, and to ascertain what is diverse and universal about human care. The goal of the theory is to use care knowledge as a guide for quality-based nursing care practices that are culturally congruent so that care will lead to health and well-being or to facing death or disability. The theory focuses not only on individual clients but also on families, groups, institutions, communities, and cultures. In contrast, Nightingale focused on the sick patient and the nurse and on health, nature, and environment. Cultural care practices were not the focus of Nightingale's views of nursing. Her goal was to have nurses place the sick patient in the best condition for nature to act on him or her by primarily providing a physical environment conducive to the reparative process.

The theory of Culture Care is extremely broad in scope. The concept of culture was derived from anthropology and the concept of human care from nursing. The two major constructs were synthesized with predictions about the universality and diversity of culture care. Culture care focuses on the *total lifeways of human beings*, with their caring expressions, values, and patterns. The theory includes world view; philosophic orientation; social structure factors such as religion, kinship, culture values, economics, education, and technology; and pays attention to language use, environmental contexts, and ethnohistory. In addition, the theory focuses on *generic* (indigenous or local folk) *care* and *professional care* values and practices in different health or community systems. These multiple factors are believed to influence care patterns and practices, which are predicted to influence the health or well-being of those being cared for or about. Moreover, these epistemic sources of care knowledge are studied and used to provide nursing care decisions and actions with three predicted modes of care: *culture care preservation or maintenance, culture care accommodation or negotiation, and culture care repatterning or restructuring*. The goal of the theory is to provide culturally congruent nursing care that is beneficial, satisfying, and leads to client health or well-being.

Culture Care theory further contrasts with Nightingale's focus on *health, nature, and environment* in that the central focus of my theory is on *human care/caring as the essence of nursing* and as the *dominant, central, and unifying domain of the discipline and profession of nursing.* Using ethnonursing research methods, the researcher can identify and document the informant's culturally-based human care components such as the support, assistance, enabling acts and other care phenomena. Nursing care decisions and actions are based on the cultural care values, beliefs, and lifeways of people in their natural or special living environment.

In using the theory of Culture Care the nurse researcher makes repeated observations and participates in the client's familiar activities or special events to identify, understand, and provide knowledge and make sound nursing care decisions—those that are tailored to fit the client's culture so that care will be meaningful and promote health and well-being. Cultures and human care/caring are extremely complex and tend to vary transculturally, hence nurses must enter the world of the people and study their care patterns, similar to the way anthropologists grasp the world of strange or unknown cultures. Culture Care theory, with its use of the ethnonursing qualitative research method, enables the nurse–researcher to discover embedded care practices in the social structure and world view by largely inductive and naturalistic participant–observation methods.

Most important, the theory is worldwide in scope yet the nurse can focus on any particular person, family, institution, community, or specific culture to document and derive knowledge that will be practical and lead to culturally congruent nursing care. Nightingale did not focus on the cultural or the meanings and patterns of human care.

Nightingale and I both focused on the importance of environment. Nightingale tended to emphasize the external physical environment as influencing and affecting the restorative process with nature, whereas I focused on environmental context as the *totality of the client's lived experiences,* including material (physical) and nonmaterial (spiritual and other social structure and world view) dimensions. Thus, the environmental context in the theory of Culture Care is far more comprehensive and includes psychophysical, sociocultural, language, ethnohistorical, and environmental contexts. Abstract and practical aspects of environment are also included.

Both my theory of nursing and Nightingale's beliefs are concerned with health, but in different ways. I view human care or care processes as *influencing health or well-being* with differences and similarities across cultures, whereas Nightingale viewed health as letting *nature act on the sick patient with the nurse providing a physical environment* conducive to the reparative process. My theory draws on such diverse culture care constructs as comfort and succor, derived from each culture as the means to health or well-being or to face death, chronic illness, or disability, whereas Nightingale draws on nature and environment to restore a patient's health.

Both Nightingale and I were bold risk-takers willing to provide breakthroughs to improve and advance nursing education, research, and practice. We share the leadership qualities of persevering over time to achieve current and future goals, risk-taking, and believing that medicine and nursing are two different but complimentary disciplines and professions. Nightingale traveled during her professional career, notably her harrowing experiences in the Crimean War as a lone nurse leader; I became the first professional nurse in the early 1960s to study human caring from a transcultural and anthropologic perspective by living with and studying the headhunters of the Eastern Highlands of New Guinea. As the only nurse to have spent two years living entirely alone with these headhunters, my experiences were probably as harrowing and equally as hectic as Nightingale's. We both survived our experiences, learned from them, and became strong leaders, carving new pathways for nursing knowledge and practice.

Finally, I must add that since the publication of *Notes on Nursing*, a number of outstanding nurse researchers, scholars, and leaders have been active to advance nursing. It is especially encouraging to see human care explicated as the central and major phenomena to understand, explain, and predict nursing. As Watson states (1985), human care is a moral imperative because it is so essential to the nature and *modus operandi* of nursing. It must continue to be studied as a transcultural phenomenon to understand human growth, development, wellness, health, and survival. We still have much to learn about human *caring* with respect to people, families, institutions, communities, and cultures. To apply such care research findings to advance nursing as a discipline is also a creative challenge. I contend that the theoretical and systematic research study of human care from a transcultural nursing perspective has been one of the most significant and distinct contributions to nursing in the 20th century. I also believe that there are other outstanding major leaders in nursing that have the potential to be equal to or even greater than Nightingale. We have, indeed, come a long way since Nightingale's time, but Nightingale was a great leader who gave new direction to nurses and nursing as a recognized, valued profession. We are most grateful for and continue to acknowledge her pioneering contributions to nursing.

REFERENCES.

Aamodt, A. (1978). Sociocultural dimensions of caring in the world of the Papago child and adolescent. In M. Leininger (Ed.), *Transcultural nursing: Concepts, theories, and practices*. New York: John Wiley & Sons.

Gaut, D. (1981). Conceptual analysis of caring: Research method. In M. Leininger (Ed.), *Caring: An essential human need* (pp. 17–24). Thorofare, NJ: Slack. (Reprinted 1988. Detroit, MI: Wayne State University Press.)

Leininger, M. (1970). *Nursing and anthropology: Two worlds to blend.* New York: John Wiley & Sons.

Leininger, M. (1977). The phenomenon of caring: The essence and central focus of nursing. *Nursing Research Report, 12* (1), 2–14.

Leininger, M. (1978). *Transcultural nursing: Concepts, theories, and practices*. New York: John Wiley & Sons

Leininger, M. (1981). *Caring: An essential human need*. Thorofare, NJ: Slack. (Reprinted 1988. Detroit, MI: Wayne State University Press.)

Leininger, M. (1984). *Care: The essence of nursing and health*. Thorofare, NJ: Slack. (Reprinted 1988. Detroit. MI: Wayne State University Press.)

Leininger, M. (1988). Leininger's theory of nursing: Cultural care diversity and universality. *Nursing Science Quarterly, 2*(4), 11–20.

Leininger, M. (1991). *Culture care diversity and universality: A theory of nursing*. New York: National League for Nursing.

Luna, L. (1989). Transcultural nursing care of Arab Muslims. *Journal of Transcultural Nursing, 1*(1), 220–227.

Nightingale, F. (1859). *Notes on nursing: What it is, and what it is not*. London: Harrison & Sons.

Orem, D. (1980). *Nursing: Concepts of practice*. New York: McGraw-Hill Book Co.

Stasiak, D. (1991). Culture care theory with Mexican-Americans in an urban context. In M. Leininger (Ed.), *Culture care diversity and universality: A theory of nursing* (pp. 179–202). New York: National League for Nursing.

Watson, J. (1979). *Nursing: The philosophy and science of caring*. Boston, MA: Little, Brown, & Co.

Watson, J. (1985). *Nursing: Human science and human care: A theory of nursing*. Norwalk, CT: Appleton-Century-Crofts.

Wenger, F. (1991). The culture care theory and the old-order Amish. In M. Leininger (Ed.). *Culture care diversity and universality: A theory of nursing* (pp. 147–178). New York: National League for Nursing.

NIGHTINGALE REDUX.

Myra Estrin Levine

It was said that the black silk tie we wore with our student uniforms was a badge of mourning for Florence Nightingale. An idealized bust of Nightingale stood at the front entrance of the Nurses' Residence. And when we had successfully completed our probationary period, we were rewarded with an organdy cap (also known as one's dignity) and a small ceramic replica of the lady's lamp. It had, after all, been a mere 30 years since her death.

Few historical figures are as victimized by their legends as she has been. The image of her as an ethereal wisp, floating among the sick, injured, and dying soldiers hovers over all the events of her life. But she was never a gentle ghost. And though she stepped into the 20th century, she was, above all, the Eminent Victorian Strachey (1918) labeled her.

The actual legacy of Victorian nursing was the rigid nurses' training I endured 50 years ago. Bound as we were by the procedure orientation and the restrictive rules of the procedure book, little space was left for personalizing patient care. The student was judged by an "Efficiency:" the meticulous performance of the written rule, step by step. The rules governing behavior were no less restrictive. The School of Nursing was a Victorian oasis and Nightingale was its guardian spirit. I was in awe of her.

As a graduate student, I was bold enough to title an essay "Nursing: What It Has Been and What It Can Be" (Levine, 1962) and I devoted the first chapter to Florence Nightingale. While writing it, I was fortunate to have access to two collections of

Myra Estrin Levine, R.N., M.S.N., D.H.L, F.A.A.N., is Professor Emerita from the College of Nursing, University of Illinois at Chicago, Chicago, Illinois.

items from Nightingale's life: the Otto Schmidt collection at Wayne State University and the Karl Meyer collection at the Cook County School of Nursing. Neither had major items, but there were her handwritten notes listing the supplies she required at Scutari and one informing her physician that he had permission to visit her at 2 p.m. that afternoon. It is difficult to describe the excitement of holding those notes, knowing that she had done so as well. And the breathless adoration is reflected in my chapter. I wrote in celebration of its message of the "heroism of that gesture which flung open the drapes and the windows to let sunshine and fresh air into the sickroom" (Levine, 1963). I console myself with the fact that serious scholarship only recently has been devoted to her. The publication of her letters (Sattin, 1987; Vicinus & Nergaard, 1990) is finally bringing Nightingale into focus—in her own voice.

When I was a student the Curriculum Guide specified the study of Sanitation. Each class was shepherded to the local sewage disposal and water purification plants. But the view of Sanitation that drove Nightingale's interest bore no relationship to 20th-century Sanitation methods. Her view of Sanitation was in vigorous conflict with her contemporaries, and it is important not merely because she was devoted to fresh air and sunshine, but because she believed poor Sanitation was the cause of all disease. Nightingale has often been gently chided for refusing to believe the germ theory. The problem was not what she failed to believe, but what she insisted was a "received" law of nature. *Notes on Nursing* is a catalog of her notions of Sanitation. "Does God think of these things so seriously?" she asks, and describes how "...sewer air from all ill-placed sink" brought "pyaemia" to a "large private house" (p. 17). She held stubbornly to the theory of "miasmas" as the cause of illness. Her views on infection and contagion were not merely polite expressions of disdain for filth and foul odor. She was a fierce antagonist, defending her conviction that "effluvia" caused sickness, scoffing at the notion that scarlet fever results from contagion, and blaming all illness on a lack of proper hygiene. We do not read *Notes on Nursing* to be taught the rules of hygiene, nor do we expect it to instruct the 20th century on the proper importance and maintenance of cleanliness. But it is a simple fact that Nightingale's discourse on Sanitation was based on false theory, laden with superstition and error. She stubbornly preached "atmospherics" while scientific evidence of contagion was being gathered around her.

For a nurse taught to follow the procedural rule without deviation under the watchful—and sometimes baneful—eye of the "probie-chaser," discovering *Notes on Nursing* was a revelation. It had a freedom that was unique in my experience. *She* cared about fresh air and noise and the behavior of visitors, and even approved of a "small pet animal" in the sickroom (p. 58).

She never wrote a text for nurses, however. The reader of *Notes on Nursing* is forewarned. The first words of the preface say:

> *The following notes are by no means intended as a rule of thought by which nurses teach themselves to nurse, still less as a manual to teach nurses to nurse (p. 1).*

She addressed the women who have "personal charge of the health of others." Its purpose was to teach "every day sanitary knowledge, or the knowledge of nursing..."(p. 1). *Notes on Nursing* is a primer on Sanitation for the women of England.

There is a deceptive immediacy in the language of *Notes on Nursing* that speaks to modern nurses a century later. As skewed as her view of the Sanitation issue was, *Notes on Nursing* displays her remarkable insight into the feelings and responses of the patient. I quoted her words on "observation" in my text (Levine, 1973), and emphasized, as I believe she did, that observation was a guardian activity. She cautioned that "it must never be lost sight of what observation is for. It is not for the sake of piling up miscellaneous information or curious facts, but for the sake of saving life and increasing health and comfort" (p. 70). The Conservation model insists that the person can only be understood in the context of environment. It emphasizes that the environment is not a passive stage setting, but rather that the person is an active participant, exploring, seeking, and testing understanding of the world he or she inhabits. The nurse cannot enter another person's environment without becoming an essential factor in it.

The nursing that Nightingale describes fits comfortably into the Conservation principles. She details the parameters of the conservation of energy. The need for fresh air, appropriate warmth, nourishing food that is suitable for the person's condition, and even "...whatever a patient *can* do for himself, it is better...for him to do for himself..." (p. 22). She cautions against over-exertion and warns that the nurse must forswear those activities that would burden the patient. "It is incredible," she says, "that nurses cannot picture to themselves the strain upon the heart, the lungs, and the brain which the act of moving is to any feeble patient" (p. 29). Many of the rules for the behavior of the nurse in the sickroom focus on the toll they take on the patient. She deplores noise—unnecessary noise places a burden on the sick, even if the noise is not loud. And she warns against waking a patient "intentionally or accidently," calling it "a *sine qua non* of all good nursing" (p. 25). The words of the 19th century make sense to the modern nurse because they speak of experiences common to the practice of nursing.

Although her physiology is very limited, Nightingale recognizes the importance of conservation of structural integrity. Her discussion of disease as a reparative process is certainly directed at the healing process, even though the rationale she provides makes no sense to the modern reader. But she knows full well what the nurse must do to bring healing. She writes, "If a patient is cold, if a patient is feverish, if a patient is faint, if he is sick after taking food, if he has a bed-sore, it is generally the fault not of the disease, but of the nursing" (p. 6). Most of her discussion of structure is related to the architecture of the hospital and the home because she believed such factors caused disease. Her battle over the architecture of St. Thomas Hospital was typical of the ferocity with which she pursued her belief. The new St. Thomas was built from 1868 to 1871 "...according to her theories of ventilation and the pavilion principle which she had always advocated and which (Sir John) Simon, with a justice endorsed by suffering posterity, condemned as unnecessary, inconvenient and grossly extravagant" (Lambert, p. 483).

Those injunctions in *Notes on Nursing* that describe the experience of the patient seem very personal, even though her own invalidism had hardly begun. She lists many of the behaviors basic to the personal integrity of the patient and the nurse. What on superficial reading appear to be small acts of kindness actually underscore the privacy and integrity of the person. She describes as a "greater worry" the cost for those who "have to endure...the incurable hopes of their friends." And she asks that the "medical attendant tell the truth to the sick..." (p. 54). She asks the nurse to "distinguish between the idiosyncrasies of patients" (p. 66). And throughout *Notes on Nursing* she identifies the importance of the person, indeed "for the well as for the sick" (p. 6).

Notes on Nursing was directed at the social integrity, health, and well-being of the English people. This was a text that was intended to describe everyday sanitary knowledge. If the nurse would care for the health of her family, "how valuable would be the produce of her united experience if every woman would think how to nurse" (p. 1).

Florence Nightingale was not a saint, merely a gifted and dedicated woman whose times and trials help us to understand our own with fresher insights. As the years increase our distance from her, she may finally be seen more as the heroic person she really was and less as the mythic heroine we have made her. This slim volume will always be a reminder to nurses everywhere of the blessing her life has placed on nursing.

REFERENCES.

Levine, M. E. (1962). *Nursing: What it has been and what it can be.* Unpublished master's essay, Wayne State University, Detroit, MI.

Lambert, R. (1963). *Sir John Simon, 1816–1904 and English social administration.* London: Macgibbon and Kee.

Levine, M. E. (1963). Florence Nightingale—The legend that lives. *Nursing Forum, 2*(4), 25–35.

Levine, M. E. (1973). *Introduction to clinical nursing* (2nd ed.). Philadelphia: F.A. Davis.

Nightingale, F. (1859). *Notes on nursing: What it is, and what it is not.* London: Harrison & Sons.

Sattin, A. (1987). *Letters from Egypt, a journey on the Nile, 1849–1850; Florence Nightingale.* New York: Weidenfeld and Nicolson.

Strachey, L. (1918), *Eminent Victorians.* New York: Modern Library edition.

Vicinus, M., & Nergaard, B. (1990). *Ever yours, Florence Nightingale: Selected letters.* Cambridge: Harvard University Press.

NIGHTINGALE'S VISION OF NURSING THEORY AND HEALTH.

Margaret A. Newman

I received my first copy of Florence Nightingale's *Notes on Nursing* as a gift from my college roommate early in our undergraduate education experience. I was impressed with its relevance then. I am even more impressed with it now. I am honored to have this opportunity to salute Nightingale for her vision regarding the development of the discipline of nursing. Her wisdom influenced my early thinking on nursing theory development in general, as well as the direction of my particular theory regarding health and patterning.

Nightingale's views on health, person–environment interaction in relation to health, and the nurse's place in facilitating health set the direction for nursing knowledge development. Retrospective analyses of nursing theory development during the past two decades have illustrated how Nightingale, as early as 1859, established the essential parameters of nursing knowledge (Newman, 1972; 1983). The key concepts set forth by Nightingale—nurse, person, environment, health—have emerged as essential interactive ingredients in nursing theory. During the past three decades the primary emphasis in theory development has been the interactive nature of nursing practice: the patient in interaction with the environment, the nurse in interaction with the patient and environment, and how these interactions facilitate the patient's health. Theorist–researchers have pointed to the unitary nature of the nursing phenomenon (Newman, Sime, & Corcoran-Perry, 1991).

Margaret A. Newman, Ph.D., R.N., F.A.A.N., is Professor of Nursing in the School of Nursing, University of Minnesota, Minneapolis, Minnesota.

Three themes in Florence Nightingale's *Notes on Nursing* have been particularly relevant to my work on health and patterning. First, her vision of nursing knowledge as *health* knowledge established health as central to a theory of nursing. Second, her characterization of disease as a reparative process foreshadowed my explication of disease as a meaningful manifestation of health. And third, her recognition of the importance of timing in the activities of nurses in relation to the rhythmic variations of patients can be seen as recognition of the importance of individual patterning in health.

Nightingale equated the knowledge of nursing with the knowledge of health.

> *I believe...that the very elements of nursing are all but unknown...are as little understood for the well as for the sick. The same laws of health or of nursing, for they are in reality the same, obtain among the well as among the sick (p. 6).*

Although my early education in nursing centered on knowledge of disease, its treatment, and how nursing relates to these factors, I was discontented with this emphasis and sought to identify and develop knowledge aimed at health, what Nightingale referred to as "the positive of which pathology is the negative" (p. 74). This search to understand the concepts of health and illness led me through the concepts of dynamic equilibrium (Johnson, 1961), stress (Selye, 1956), high-level wellness (Dunn, 1959), and finally to a shift in viewing the process as a unidirectional process of increasing complexity (Rogers, 1970). Health emerged as the synthesis of wellness and illness, as the evolving pattern of the whole (Newman, 1979; 1986).

Second, Nightingale's apparent polarization of health and disease cannot be taken literally, since she also stated clearly in the opening sentence of her book that *disease is a reparative process.*

> *Shall we begin by taking it as a general principle—that all disease...is more or less a reparative process...an effort of nature to remedy a process...(p. 5).*

This premise is inherent in my theory of health as expanding consciousness. An assumption of my theory is that the pattern of life evolves through periods of order and disorder in a unidirectional manner to higher levels of consciousness. The disorder may be equated with what we label disease. Efforts to restore the equilibrium of the previous stage of order fail to recognize the disorder as part of the evolving pattern. Such an action may deter the organism's natural movement to higher levels of organization, consciousness, and health. When disease is present, it is regarded as a necessary part of the self-organizing process of the living system to higher levels of organization—a reparative process.

The third point I would like to address is Nightingale's foresight in recognizing *timing* in the attention to variation in patients' responses to environmental input. She emphasized the importance of

...consulting the hours when the patient can take food, the observation of the times, often varying, when he is most faint, the altering seasons of taking food...

I have known a patient's life saved...by the simple question..."But is there no hour when you feel you could eat?" "Oh, yes," he said, "I could always take something at ___ o'clock and ___ o'clock" (p. 37).

Serious study of biologic rhythms has been underway since the 1960s, only about 25 years. Application of this knowledge to nursing has received cursory attention. Some of the research that has found its way into nursing practice involves variations in personal space needs, learning and performance abilities, receptivity to drug therapy, and individual openness to interpersonal activity. Unfortunately today the examples of violations of patients' temporal patterns within acute-care centers outweigh the application of sensitivity to these needs. There are examples coming to light in a broader sense of the importance of timing in relationships, however. Nurse case managers attest to the importance of sensitivity to the timing of visits in the effectiveness of their interactions in meeting the clients' needs (Newman, Lamb, & Michaels, 1991). Nightingale sensed over 100 years ago the importance of recognizing a patient's temporal patterns in providing effective care.

Finally, Nightingale made it clear that nurses were not born but educated, so that they would be able to *"think* how to nurse" (emphasis added) (p. 1). Educators, theorist–researchers, and practitioners owe a tremendous debt to the vision Nightingale had for the nature of nursing knowledge and practice. It is fitting that we celebrate a revival of her notes on nursing.

REFERENCES.

Dunn, H. L. (1959). High level wellness for man and society. *American Journal of Public Health*, *49*, 786–792.

Johnson, D. (1961). The significance of nursing care. *American Journal of Nursing*, *61*(11), 63–66.

Newman, M. A. (1972). Nursing's theoretical evolution. *Nursing Outlook*, *20*(7), 449–453.

Newman, M. A. (1979). *Theory development in nursing*. Philadelphia: F.A. Davis.

Newman, M. A. (1983). The continuing revolution: A history of nursing science. In N. L. Chaska (Ed.), *The nursing profession: A time to speak* (pp. 385–393). New York: McGraw-Hill.

Newman, M. A. (1986). *Health as expanding consciousness.* St. Louis: C.V. Mosby.

Newman, M. A., Lamb, G. S., & Michaels, C. (1991). Nurse case management: The coming together of theory and practice. *Nursing and Health Care, 12*(8), 404–408.

Newman, M. A., Sime, A. M., & Corcoran-Perry, S. A. (1991). The focus of the discipline of nursing. *Advances in Nursing Science, 14*(1), 1–6.

Nightingale, F. (1859). *Notes on nursing: What it is, and what it is not.* London: Harrison & Sons.

Rogers, M. E. (1970). *An introduction to the theoretical basis of nursing.* Philadelphia: F.A. Davis.

Selye, H. (1956). *The stress of life.* New York: McGraw-Hill.

NOTES ON NIGHTINGALE.

Hildegard E. Peplau

The roots of nursing lie deep in human history. One notable marker in nursing's progress toward becoming a profession is Florence Nightingale's book, *Notes on Nursing,* published in 1859.

This book can best be understood as a period piece, a reflection of commonly held views about women and Nightingale's conceptions of nursing at the mid-19th century. She asserts that "a nurse means any person in charge of the personal health of another" (p. 79). The book is addressed to "everywoman" and to nurses. By this means, Nightingale affirmed a traditionally held link between the long, historical role of women at home and in the community, and the practices of nurses in her time and place. I wondered how Nightingale reconciled this commonly held notion with her drive to establish "training schools" for the preparation of selected women for a "calling" into nursing (p. 63). Furthermore, she decries practices of "amateur females" (p. 73). Today the idea that "everywoman" is a nurse applies only in an exceedingly limited way as the extraordinary and increasing complexity of professional nursing is being recognized. Nightingale's attribution of nursing also excluded men. In earlier centuries there were religious and military orders in which men engaged in nursing. This failure to recognize male nurses is still evident in the slow recruitment of men into the contemporary profession of nursing. Nightingale was a product of her era and did not envision the possibility of changing roles and relationships between women and men.

Hildegard E. Peplau, R.N., Ed.D., F.A.A.N., is Professor Emerita, Rutgers, The State University of New Jersey, Newark, New Jersey.

Mental illness was not uncommon in Nightingale's day—there were asylums in England in the 19th century. Nightingale did not consider nursing practiced in these institutions in her published works.

Nightingale was influenced by some of the great ideas of her time. She was educated and well read. It is conceivable that ideas commonly being debated in Victorian society were also discussed among her friends and acquaintances within the elite group to which the Nightingale family belonged. Among the constructs to emerge in the 1800s were the natural order of things, natural selection (Darwin), and germ theory (Pasteur). Nightingale emphasized "Nature" and "nature," apparently ignored Darwin, and rejected Pasteur's germ theory. Her definitions and descriptions of nursing reflect these choices.

Nightingale was also affected by her home environment. The Nightingale home was surely among the great manor houses of England. Such homes tended to have an "upstairs–downstairs" ambiance, with the household managed by a matron who supervised staff in matters of light, cleanliness, order, punctuality, and so forth. These concerns also appear in Nightingale's descriptions of nursing practice.

Nightingale described nursing as "how to put the constitution in such a state as that it will have no disease..."(p. 1). This statement can be rephrased as, "What can and should nurses do to promote health, prevent illness, and aid recovery from disease?" Contemporary nurses generally accept this restatement; however, Nightingale's descriptions of nursing practice do not specifically show relationships between nursing actions and the state of the "constitution" of the person receiving nursing care. The book includes comments on the prevention of complications during illness but little is said about prevention of disease. She opposed vaccination for smallpox.

Moreover, Nightingale's elaboration of the definition, which she called a "principle," is rather curious. Diseases are called a "reparative process...which Nature has instituted" in an effort to "remedy a process of poisoning or of decay," of short or long duration (p. 5). This would seem to put nursing in opposition to Nature (God?); both fix things that are lacking, but nurses do it better. The symptoms of disease and suffering, according to Nightingale, were due to lacks or " the want of fresh air, or of light, or of warmth, or of quiet, or of cleanliness, or of punctuality (regarding diet)" (pp. 5–6). Nightingale does not clarify her intended use of the term Nature but the impression is easily gained that when the word is spelled with a capital "N" it is synonymous with God. She was a deeply religious person.

Notes on Nursing is primarily about the conduct and practices of nurses. It describes what nurses do or should do and some patient dilemmas, but it skirts discussion of nurse–patient interactions or relationships. For instance, patients who are worried by "ghosts of their troubles" are to get relief from "their anxieties" from "variety," the nurse being advised to move the bed so that the patient can look out the window (p. 35). Patients did not want to talk about themselves, she said (p. 55). Nightingale emphasized teaching nurses what and how to observe (p. 59). She had strong words about visitors and nurses giving advice or trying to cheer up patients, stating that it was generally injurious (p. 57). The "handicraft of nursing" (p. 71) supported the "natural processes of health" (p. 53) by abiding by the "laws of health" (p. 79) pertaining to provision of light, fresh air, and so forth.

The foregoing critique notwithstanding, and given that the ideas are over one century old and bound by the era in which Nightingale lived and worked, they do invite thought and had some bearing on my own professional work.

My introduction to Nightingale was by way of the nurse's pledge that bears her name. It was etched deeply in my mind as a consequence of repetition required by my teachers in "training school," when I was a student nurse from 1928 to 1931. A brief sketch of Nightingale's life and work was presented in a class or two on the history of nursing. She was portrayed as the leader of modern nursing.

A very large part of what I was taught as nursing practice had to do with the essentials described in *Notes on Nursing*. For example, when caring for pneumonia patients, I spent long hours, day and night, wrapped in blankets, sitting next to windows open in winter to provide fresh air for patients who were kept warm by their high fevers, many blankets, and hot water bottles. I scrubbed and fumigated rooms, carbolized beds, and sterilized equipment all in the interest of cleanliness. And woe unto student nurses in the diet kitchen, where they prepared and cooked all food for patients, if the diet trays were late being put onto the dumbwaiter and if, after signalling, the ropes of pulleys were not pulled to transport them up to the patient floors in the hospital on time. Talking with patients was considered both a waste of time and possibly a dangerous intrusion into the domain of physicians—or worse, "getting personal" with patients, which was considered unethical.

My next contact with the "lady with the lamp" was at Teachers College, Columbia University. In 1948 I was invited to return to Teachers College, where I had completed a Master of Arts degree in 1947, to join the psychiatric nursing program that had been started in 1945. The program as I had experienced it was a hodgepodge of visiting lecturers, visits to clinical sites, and a brief clinical practicum. There were also inspiring nursing courses taught by such illustrious nursing leaders as Isabel Stewart and Elizabeth Burgess, as well as required nonnursing courses. Stewart and Burgess often referred to the great work of Nightingale.

In 1948, as instructor and director of the graduate program in psychiatric nursing, my immediate task was to design and provide a psychiatric nursing educative experience that would be a vast improvement over the one I had had. My duty to the profession, as I saw it, was to gain recognition for the program as reputable graduate-level education. Furthermore, the program was expected to produce leaders in psychiatric nursing who were knowledgeable and competent in clinical practice, teaching, and supervision—all in one academic year. When I approached this formidable task I had only my baccalaureate education at Bennington College and some earlier unusually rich, clinically educative experiences for background assistance. At the first Nursing Division faculty meeting, I was also named chair of the "definition of nursing committee"—I was the only member and this was my only committee assignment.

To prepare for the work ahead I first headed to the library to seek nursing definitions. Another aim was to review all of the available textbooks on psychiatric nursing, select the most relevant content, in my judgment, and design appropriate course work. This endeavor was not as fruitful as I anticipated. What was most obvious in these textbooks was the preponderance of "ought," "should," and "must" terms regarding what nurses were to do *to* or *for* patients, with no clear statements as to when or why the actions were to be taken or how they might prove beneficial to patients. Meanwhile, graduate students were registering for admission to the program. I came upon some of Nightingale's work during my search and allowed myself to get partially sidetracked into reviewing the Nightingale collection. At the same time I was also searching the psychiatric and social science literature to prepare for the nursing courses I had to teach, along with making arrangements for the students' clinical work.

At that time Teachers College had a substantial collection of Nightingale papers, memorabilia, and some published biographies. These were easily accessible; I actually held some originals many times. I became so intrigued that I even wrote a paper comparing some of Nightingale's ideas with those of other thinkers of her time. Isabel Stewart, to whom I showed the paper, was not impressed and asked me never to publish it. The paper was not required for course work so it simply got filed.

Nevertheless, when reading Nightingale's *Notes on Nursing,* I came upon her definition of nursing (p. 1) and her various references to "the reparative process" that "Nature has instituted" (p. 5). These constructs caught my attention. I puzzled over her statement that "what nursing has to do...is to put the patient in the best condition for nature to act upon him" (p. 75). (Note that "nature" here is in lower case, so in this sentence she doesn't refer to God but perhaps to something within the person.) To try to grasp what Nightingale's covert meaning might have been, I reframed her statement many different ways to reflect possible hidden meanings. I may also have gone beyond it to interject my view, which was then evolving, of what nursing was, should, or could be. For example, I came up with such rephrasings as:

• The work of nurses is to support the person's processes of bodily repair until the functional bodily processes are restored and begin to function fully again; or
• Nurses support the person's functional bodily processes in some way until their normal functions are restored.

These restatements clearly differ from Nightingale's views. She saw disease as a reparative process and symptoms of disease as not always the cause (p. 5), but as due to lacks or "wants" of fresh air and so on. I was then thinking in terms of either separate processes of bodily repair or dysfunctional bodily processes. And I considered symptoms not as "causes," perhaps due to "lacks" or "wants," but surely as cues to bodily dysfunction for some reason—that is, as human responses to diseases or dysfunctional bodily processes due to a cause that could be identified and explained.

In *Notes on Nursing*, Nightingale does not specifically identify the bodily processes in question. For example, in discussing the rule "to keep the air within as pure as the air without" (p. 8), she does not relate this nursing action to the respiratory process. Nor does she describe how pure air would support and thus begin a reparative process. Similarly, she does not point to the digestive or eliminative processes in relation to taking food (pp. 36–44). As a student nurse in 1929, one of the questions I encountered on a written examination for a course taught by a physician was to "describe the path of the ingestion of a ham sandwich as it passes through the digestive and eliminative systems." I never forgot the question; it came to mind easily when first reading *Notes on Nursing* many years ago.

Nightingale's failure to specify processes is not a shortcoming, but rather a reflection of limited knowledge of these matters. Moreover, she states and describes what nurses do—the activities they performed in hospitals in her day. Most of these activities were subsequently contained in popular definitions of nursing up until 1970. That was when the New York State Nurses Association achieved a major change in the definition of nursing in the New York Nursing Practice Act. This Act states that nurses "diagnose and treat" and it pinpoints a phenomenologic focus for nursing practice. This new definition is described in the American Nurses Association report, *Nursing: A Social Policy Statement* (1980).

Nightingale's definition set me to thinking about bodily processes: what they were, how they worked, and how nurses of my day supported them without using invasive procedures or medications. I knew both firsthand and analytically, for example, the intended purposes served by the external application of poultices to infected boils or to the chests of pneumonia patients. I knew the nursing action of pouring water from a pitcher into a bucket so that the sound might stimulate urinary output. There were other such nursing practices mostly derived from folkways that are now considered quaint and outmoded.

At one point I made a list of bodily processes and began a literature search on what was known scientifically about their function and dysfunction, in the hope of eventually formulating a supportive regimen that might be considered for nursing practice. But psychiatric nursing rather than medical-surgical nursing required my full attention, and this interesting intellectual venture was put aside. I did discuss this interest often with nurses then teaching or practicing in medical-surgical nursing, however, in the hope that someone else would pursue this line of inquiry. I even arranged a summer workshop at Teachers College for nurse-science teachers from across the country to consider what scientific principles and concepts were defined as and relate them to functions of bodily processes.

In 1949 I submitted the manuscript for my book, *Interpersonal Relations in Nursing,* to a publisher who offered to publish it if I added a physician as first author, a proposal I immediately rejected. G.P. Putnam published the book in 1952. (It was reissued in 1991 by Springer Publishing Co.) Putnam had a nurse committee that reviewed the manuscript and made suggestions such as "take this out," "put this in," "you shouldn't say this," and so delayed its publication. The nurses' names do not appear in the book at their request. This vignette is included only to illustrate that anxiety ran high with publishers and nurses, suggesting that the ideas in the manuscript were indeed a radical departure from the conceptions of nursing at that time. It was a nonnurse, Genevieve Bixler, who advised Putnam to "Publish it!"

In that book I defined nursing as an interpersonal, educative, and therapeutic process. I said that "nursing is to function in cooperation with internal and external human processes" and that to do that, it was "necessary to have knowledge of particular processes and of their relationship to the solution of specific interpersonal problems" (Peplau, p. 13). My interest in processes, particularly those relevant to competent practices of psychiatric nurses, arose from reframing Nightingale's definition.

In a quarter century of graduate-level teaching in psychiatric nursing, I pursued an interest in explanatory constructs—concepts and processes. The search was for theoretical constructs that nurses could apply to understand the observations they were making during interactions with psychiatric patients. In the late 1940s the only patients public mental hospital administrators allowed graduate nurse students to interview and study were chronic patients, some of whom had been hospitalized for 40 years. It was thought that nurses could do them no harm. Their psychopathology, including hallucinations and delusions, was evident. Their anxiety was pervasive and ever-present. I made the assumption that a theoretical explanation of these presenting phenomena could be used to derive verbal nursing interventions. Such actions, if sustained over time, would evoke beneficial outcomes for the patients. This approach was clearly different from the practical, "everywoman" actions described in *Notes on Nursing*. At first I often had doubts about the direction I was taking. In 1948, I saw Isabel Stewart in the halls of Teachers College and told her of my appointment. She said, "I do hope that you are being practical." Her comment crossed my mind often thereafter. At first nurse colleagues and even some of the graduate students objected vehemently to helping patients to become aware of feeling anxious (O'Toole & Welt, 1989, p. 281) or to begin to understand their need for the hallucinatory process (O'Toole & Welt, 1989, p. 311). The prevailing nursing approach then, as in *Notes on Nursing*, was to avoid these matters and change the subject.

In the Teachers College and Rutgers programs, which I directed, the emphasis of faculty and graduate students was on knowing and using theoretical constructs and formulating new ones from clinical data. Briefly, at first the focus was on intrapersonal processes (as in the work of Freud), then on interpersonal processes (as in the work of H.S. Sullivan), then on systems processes (such as the work of von Bertalanffy), and finally on family systems processes (including the work of Jay Haley and others). Out of these efforts came a theory-based practice of psychiatric nursing.

Nursing in Nightingale's time was activity-oriented. Nursing practice was described as what a nurse can, or should, do *to* or *for* patients. What is missing are relationships between the action to be taken and the need for it in terms of the patient's condition, and the effect the action is intended to produce on that condition. There is little in *Notes on Nursing* about problems, needs, or concerns of patients as described by them. There is much on what nurses are to do, most of it focused on the environment—keeping it clean, quiet, well-lit, and freshly aired. The focus is largely on rules, duties, activities, and "proper conduct" that nurses are to maintain.

The shift toward interpersonal theory was pivotal. Its emphasis on nurse–patient relations and theoretical constructs to explain patient dilemmas was new to nursing. The effort to derive nursing actions from theory and consider their intended corrective effects on patient problems was substantially different from Nightingale's framework. The shift also deemphasized spectator observation, that is, nurses observing patients as objects. Instead it emphasized participant-observation, with the nurse observing herself, the other, and the relationships occurring in the interaction.

Theory-based nursing practice is a new paradigm. It emerged just after World War II and gained impetus within the nursing profession in the 1950s, a century after Nightingale's *Notes on Nursing* first appeared. The timing of this new direction for nursing was fortuitous. It corresponded to a rapid evolution of medical science and technology, which spawned many unforeseen changes in hospital care. Early ambulation, for instance, heralded a decline in widespread use of traditional bedside nursing care and the development of new requirements for nurses. Sophisticated technology and a wide array of pharmaceuticals were unknown in Nightingale's day. The new paradigm also coincided with an explosion of knowledge in all fields, especially in both basic and applied sciences. Another major factor that required and supported theory-based nursing was the rise of academic-based nursing education, and particularly the development of graduate-level nursing education programs. These began to replace hospital-based postgraduate courses in the 1940s.

The shift from an activity orientation, with its focus on what nurses do, to a knowledge-based nursing practice, emphasizing what nurses know theoretically and use intellectually to design and guide nursing practice, was a timely occurrence. In effect, the climate of the changing times required it. Similarly, Nightingale's efforts and their subsequent impact on nursing were coincident with great social changes in her time—the Industrial Revolution, the rapid rise of hospitals and the need to make them clean and safe, and the emerging need for more nurses to provide a supply for a growing demand.

Some of Nightingale's ideas in *Notes on Nursing* are fuzzy, to say the least, and some are outmoded. It was her first book, and she did claim only to be giving "hints." It is unfair to judge her contribution to nursing based on one 1859 publication. I feel the same way when my 1952 first book is judged as if it were my only contribution to the profession, despite my many other publications. Even so, *Interpersonal Relations in Nursing* does lay out, in broad strokes, a new description of nursing and nurse–patient relationships quite different from that in Nightingale's book. It too is fuzzy in parts, however. It is incomplete. I can try to justify its shortcomings, which Nightingale cannot do on her own behalf, but certainly she would if she were still living.

Interpersonal Relations in Nursing defines nursing as a process and suggests the need of nurses to understand particular processes. Yet these processes are neither named, described, nor explained; the term "process" doesn't appear in the index. The process of personality development underlies the whole work. Later publications—mine and those of nurses who studied with me—contain many other theoretical constructs, including concepts and interpersonal processes that are identified and defined, for which practice applications are shown. These include but are not limited to anxiety, conflict, self-system, language–thought process, hallucinatory process, investigative counseling process, and so on (O'Toole & Welt, 1989). At Rutgers graduate students in psychiatric nursing studied in depth such processes as attention, perception, and dissociation, which are very relevant to psychiatric nursing.

The idea of processes did not first occur to me when reading Nightingale's work, which merely pointed to a term I already knew. Her book served to remind me of a construct at a time when I urgently needed to begin to use it more fully. What I do acknowledge from *Notes on Nursing* is the idea of nurses supporting "reparative processes" within the person in such a way as to enable restoration of functioning.

To me the learning process is a reparative process. It is complex. (I have defined this process elsewhere [O'Toole & Welt, 1989, pp. 348–352].) Learning is the main work of psychiatric patients. Learning is not always necessarily a consequence of teaching, but rather an effort the learner (student nurse or psychiatric patient) makes that a teacher or therapist can aid or thwart according to the practices used. Nightingale understood this point, although she didn't elaborate on it. She said of women and particularly of student nurses, "...I ask her to teach herself" using "hints" from *Notes on Nursing* (p. 1). It is a point worth knowing.

Nightingale was not a devotee of physicians, although she did not indulge in the "doctor bashing" that can occur today. She said, "...medicine is the surgery of functions, as surgery proper is that of limbs and organs. Neither can do anything but remove obstructions; neither can cure; nature alone cures" (p. 74). She also said, "...medicine, so far as we know, assists nature to remove the obstruction, but does nothing more. And what nursing has to do...is to put the patient in the best condition for nature to act upon him" (p. 75). Thus, both physicians and nurses need to understand "nature." If only Nightingale had described fully and precisely what she meant by Nature or nature!

A final point—some ideas become obsolete; their use becomes outmoded by changing social circumstances. Some ideas are timeless; they survive the tests that inevitable social changes impose on them. Ideas can be reframed, teasing out what may be a hidden meaning. Such restated ideas can be developed further, to be tested anew, in the crucible of social change and intellectual progress. This can be said of Nightingale's *Notes on Nursing*. My ideas are subject to the same judgments of history.

REFERENCES.

Nightingale, F. (1859). *Notes on nursing: What it is, and what it is not.* London: Harrison & Sons.

O'Toole, A.W., & Welt, S.R. (Eds.). (1989). *Interpersonal theory in nursing practice: Selected works of Hildegard E. Peplau.* New York: Springer Publishing Co.

Peplau, H.E. (1991). *Interpersonal relations in nursing.* New York: Springer Publishing Company. (Original work published 1952)

American Nurses Association. (1980). *Nursing: A social policy statement.* Kansas City, MO: American Nurses Association.

NIGHTINGALE'S
NOTES ON NURSING:
PRELUDE TO THE 21ST CENTURY.

Martha E. Rogers

Florence Nightingale's *Notes on Nursing* is an exciting and far-reaching compendium of ideas and statements concerning the purposes and scope of nursing, the essentials of good nursing practice, and the variety of providers of nursing that existed in her purview. With consummate skill and cogent humor she decries the fallacies in health practices and the superstitions that existed among the public and in particular health workers.

The thoughtful reader can find in *Notes on Nursing* the underpinnings for much of what is going on today. In fact, she spells out the purpose of nursing as the promotion of health and speaks to the broad scope of nursing when she notes the practices of health promotion that belong in homes, hospitals, schools, playgrounds, the workplace, the military, and all places. To this broad scope she adds emphasis on the need for fewer hospitals, not more, the differentiation of nursing practitioners, and knowledgeable nursing by educated people to direct those who are trained to function either in the home or as trained nurses.

Although she is oriented to the era in which she lived, the depth of her vision is obvious when one looks beyond the surface. The concepts of human compassion, a broad knowledge base, intelligent reasoning, and understanding not only provide a picture of what nursing needed to be in 1859 when she wrote this book, but also propose ways in which we can look at it now. As we approach the 21st century we are moving into a world that on

Martha E. Rogers, R.N., Sc.D., F.A.A.N., is Professor Emerita, New York University, New York, New York.

the surface is quite different from Nightingale's, where the need for knowledgeable nursing is increasingly in the forefront. We are moving from nursing's prescientific era into nursing's scientific era, in which an organized abstract system rooted in a new reality provides the basis for the autonomous nursing practice Nightingale emphasized. She was quite clear in noting that nurses worked with, but were not secondary to, others.

Nightingale's essentials included such things as pure air, pure water (environmentalists will note she was ahead of her time), efficient drainage, cleanliness, light, good nutrition, freedom from anxiety, and humor. A range of other factors were noted and discussed, and reasons why they were important were given. In fact, in her reasoning of the world in general and man's place in it, Nightingale brought to bear statistical evidence, logic, intellectual acumen, and vision.

Readers of *Notes on Nursing* should beware that within Nightingale's seemingly simple recommendations are many extremely significant ideas of far-reaching import. Her comments on the need for knowing observations foretell the significance of research and the study of phenomena to better understand the directions in which one might best go. Her differentiation of those who nurse into the knowledgeable and those who must take their direction from them has considerable significance when today's differences between entrance levels to nursing are considered. Nursing continues to have two entrance levels.

Nightingale emphasizes the uniqueness of nursing in terms of both the knowledge base that nurses need to possess and the nature of practice, in which nurses properly use their knowledge base *to* practice. In other words, nursing practice itself is not enough. This point is well taken, considering today's efforts to determine the nature of nursing's knowledge base within a more specific framework. Nightingale proposes that whether the person is mistress of a large country house or matron of a hospital, their need for a knowledgeable foundation and for putting this knowledge to work in the training of people to follow their directions can do a great deal to assist development of a healthy society.

As nurses continue to struggle to develop an image of nursing commensurate with the 21st century, Nightingale's words should be considered: (to be a good nurse) "...requires nothing but a disappointment in love, the want of an object, a general disgust, or incapacity for other things" (p. 75). The need for such a statement gives a very good idea of the kinds of attitudes that Nightingale faced. It is reported that Nightingale, on hearing a doctor say that the qualities of a good nurse were only that she be neat, clean, and obedient, responded that as much could be said for a good horse. The idea of a nurse as someone who is neat, clean, and obedient has not left the image market. One has only to look at some of the statements found in many different places today among nurses and others to recognize that old images have not disappeared. As the 21st century approaches identification of the uniqueness of nursing, its purpose, and its scope becomes increasingly important if nurses are to take their place among other providers in the health arena.

A spacebound society foretells the needs for a new reality and new ways of looking at people and their world. Synthesis and pattern seeing are significant aspects of this new reality. A body of knowledge specific to nursing is essential if nurses are to provide services that we purport to be assistive, which Nightingale emphasized was necessary to fulfill our responsibilities to people. As a knowledgeable endeavor the term nursing becomes a noun signifying an organized body of abstract knowledge. The practice of nursing is the imaginative use of this knowledge for human betterment. The development of this knowledge depends on research and theory development. Transmission of this knowledge takes place through the educational process. Nurses must provide knowledgeable leadership as well as be able to make judgments about clarification of career levels, just as Nightingale spoke about careers in nursing she believed were important.

Research will continue to add to this body of knowledge. As nurses seek advanced study to enable them to pursue increasing nursing knowledge, there must also be an organized abstract system specific to nursing. The practice of nursing is the creative and imaginative use of knowledge for human betterment. It is important to note that a new reality underlies nursing science and its practice.

Certainly the practice modalities advocated by Nightingale fit into noninvasive nursing practice. If one looks at what is significant today, one would not question the value of Nightingale's proposals, nor does it seem likely that the points one might add in modern language are that different from those at the time Nightingale was working. In today's language these include meditation, therapeutic touch, imagery, humor, and various other modalities, many of which are yet to come. It is relevant to draw attention to the use of caring as a way of using nursing knowledge; it should not be confused with the science of nursing. Nightingale emphasized the significant role of the environment in the healing process. Not only were the basics of clean air, light, proper nutrition, and sanitation of primary importance, but also "variety," such as a view of the outdoors, a change in surroundings, paintings, colorful flowers, plants, and music, was emphasized. She also notes that some visitors (another environmental factor) can do more harm than good and recommends that perhaps time spent with "a small pet animal" or with a young child or infant can do more to speed recovery (p. 58). These practical illustrations of Nightingale's vision continue to be valid in today's world and portray examples of use of the science of nursing.

Nightingale's identification of nursing essentials seems to continue to be of extreme importance in today's world and in the world of the future. Over-emphasis on technology tends to overshadow therapeutic modalities that can have real significance. Nurses must recognize that they do not create change in people, rather they participate in the process of change to the extent that they bring knowledge to the situation and recognize that the healing process has the potential for healing beyond that which we tend to recognize today. The answer to health will not be found in more drugs, more technology, or more hospitals.

It is remarkable the extent to which Nightingale set in motion an essential community service designed to further human health and wellbeing. Her ideas not only are meaningful today, but also provide a firm foundation as nurses move forward in the development of nursing as a science in its own right, and make way for knowledgeable direction that enables nurses to practice based on their own phenomena of concern. It is the uniqueness of nursing that makes it important, not the ways in which it is like other fields. This is a point that we need to consider carefully; Nightingale was pointing it out when she commented that medicine and nursing should never be mixed up, since it spoils both.

We live in a fantastic world. People are no longer planet-bound; rather, we are space-directed. In the next century we can expect that not only will people be living on other planets, but also the evolutionary process can be expected to promote further change that will transcend homo sapiens to coordinate with our extended understanding of space environment. The ability of nurses as well as others to comprehend the significance of this expanding universe and our role in it will be an important aspect of the nature of change, in which nurses participate in the process of working with human beings and those who will come after us.

Rogerian science of irreducible human beings provides a framework rooted in a new reality and directed toward moving us from what might be called a prescientific era to a scientific era. Certainly Nightingale laid a firm foundation for this kind of an approach to nursing knowledge and its use. The organized abstract system focuses on people and their world, which identifies the uniqueness of nursing. The primary focus of nursing is to promote health in this continually changing evolutionary process. It is from this organized abstract system that many principles and theories derive. Already these are under extensive investigation and are providing new ways of looking at things. Moreover, it seems possible that there is a tremendous push toward holistic thinking and better organization of our knowledge in the direction of new visions, including energy fields, wave phe-

nomena, and space potentials—all of which do have meaning
that we must share. As other ways of knowing are united with
earlier ideas we can expect an exciting new world to emerge.
Nurses will be an integral part of this new world.

Dr. Rogers would like to express her appreciation to Kathy Rapacz
for editorial assistance in the preparation of this manuscript.

VIGOR, VARIABLES, AND VISION: COMMENTARY ON FLORENCE NIGHTINGALE.

Sister Callista Roy

Florence Nightingale's vigor for life, belief in being able to effect change, and vision of the ideal and the real command attention throughout her writings and her work. Nightingale's notions of nursing, and the deliberative activist that she was, most forcefully presented in this historic volume, have had a deep impact on my own thinking and practice of nursing. This did not take place all at once, but grew as my own convictions and commitments matured. In several ways her message predictably presaged my own, since I am a member of the profession that she is credited with founding. Yet there is a distinct demarcation—I live in a different time and therefore have other perspectives on thought and action. I count as an advantage both that Nightingale provided such a rich heritage and that I live in this time, with the challenges of nursing at the turn of this century. Despite her disciplined and lofty image, I sometimes wish I could sit down with Nightingale and talk over her views on continuing and emerging issues in nursing; at other times I think I know exactly what she would say.

Sister Callista Roy, R.N., Ph.D., F.A.A.N., is Professor at the School of Nursing, Boston College, Chestnut Hill, Massachusetts, and is Research Professor in Nursing, Mount St. Mary's College, Los Angeles, California.

ENHANCING INNATE LIFE PROCESSES.

A key theme in Nightingale's beliefs about nursing was that it not signify merely "the administration of medicines and the application of poultices" (p. 6), but rather the knowledge of how to promote "health existences" and the proper use of the environment to aid the natural reparative processes "—all at the least expense of vital power to the patient" (p. 6). I might use different words today, but I believe my own work is congruent with this position, and in fact extends it in several ways.

As a beginning nursing student, I was struck by the 19th century belief that healing was a natural process. Nightingale noted that pain and suffering of illness were related, not to the disease, but to the absence of one or all of her stated essentials of nursing, that is, the proper use of fresh air, light, warmth, cleanliness, quiet, and the proper selection and administration of diet. Surrounded by the positivist approach of many of the sciences I studied, I became aware that phrases such as "surgery removes the bullet out of the limb...but nature heals the wound" (p. 74–75) were not entirely acceptable in scientific discussion. At the same time I was also receiving a fine liberal arts education and kept my perspective on natural processes intact through philosophy, theology, poetry, history, language, economics, sociology, anthropology, psychology, and political science. As a young staff nurse I was immediately impressed with the resilience of children in the recovery process, both from disease and from the many changes of hospitalization, with even a small amount of well-timed nursing care. Thus, my original insights into viewing the person as having innate and acquired abilities to deal with a changing environment were developed. Later I articulated this belief by using the concept of adaptation.

This concept was rich and meaningful, especially because I understood adaptation to be a dynamic process, not a return to equilibrium. My position of a later 20th century scholar gives me rich knowledge of peoples' natural processes, or life processes, as I call them. By taking a large sample of clinical situations (500 descriptions of patient behavior written by student nurses), I determined that it was reasonable to consider that adaptive processes were taking place in four domains, considered representative of clinical practice. From current literature we can understand such processes on a physiologic level and how they are manifested in self-concept, role mastery, and interdependence.

The inner dynamism for the process of adaptation I called the *regulator* and *cognator*. Nightingale noted that it was extraordinary that the education of women in her time included the elements of astronomy, given that "the laws of the motions of the heavenly bodies, far removed as they are from us, are perfectly well understood" (p. 7). Yet the "laws of the human mind, which are under our observation all day...are no better understood than they were two thousand years ago" (p. 7). Still more she decried the fact that mothers, teachers, and nurses of any class were not "taught anything about those laws which...make these bodies, into which He (God) has put our minds, healthy or unhealthy organs of those minds" (p. 7). She particularly lamented that the laws of life, as she called them, were in a certain measure understood, but not even mothers thought it worthwhile to study them and how to give their children healthy existences, rather thinking this medical or physiologic knowledge, fit only for doctors.

My own search for these "laws of life" began as a child, continued from my years in a baccalaureate program, and later intensified as a postdoctoral fellow. While in the third grade, I remember my classmates turning to me for answers to the question of whether or not other children could be allowed to lick their ice cream bars. After setting straight the fact that the various races and colors of the children in our school called for all of them to be treated the same, I then delivered a speech on the rudiments of understanding transfer of organisms. This was probably learned from my mother when helping to care for my younger brothers and sisters, since my mother studied well how to give her "children healthy existences."

Later I recall the absolute awe in discovering the wonders of the central nervous system, and the new pattern of the matter of life, DNA, that had just been discovered. Working with the Roy Adaptation Model, the regulator and cognator became my way of expressing central life processes within changing environments. An open systems model seemed most useful in conceptualizing these ideas. Although I had an additional century of human knowledge to help express my ideas, they essentially followed Nightingale's central theme. My conviction that human life processes are the core of basic nursing science and that managing the environment is the focus of clinical nursing became more explicit through the years. Eventually I became convinced of the need to do postdoctoral studies in nursing and chose the field of neuroscience nursing because of the possibilities it offered to delve deeper into knowledge of the regulator and cognator and their interrelationships in the human life process of adaptation. As with Nightingale I did not want the natural reparative processes to be interrupted by lack of knowledge. Mentored by an expert nurse/scientist, Dr. Connie Robinson, these two years more than fulfilled my hopes in further opening to me the wonders of individual adaptation through the magnificent nervous system orchestration. At the same time, this experience left me with an agenda for a lifetime—to continue to discover the laws or patterns of the innate human life processes.

EFFECTING OUTCOMES FOR
INDIVIDUALS AND SOCIETY.

A cardinal principle for Nightingale was that "the exact value of particular remedies and modes of treatment were by no means ascertained, while there is universal experience as to the extreme importance of careful nursing in determining the issue of the disease" (p. 6). Similarly, she strongly objected to the statement that "the circumstances which govern our children's healths are beyond our control" (p. 7). Nightingale established for all time the universal accountability of professional nursing. She met the challenge of whether or not any care can prevent a patient from suffering this or that with the simple response, "I humbly say, I do not know. But when you have done away with all that pain and suffering, which in patients are the symptoms not of their disease, but of the absence of one or all of the...essentials" (p. 6) of nursing care, then we will know what are the symptoms of the disease and the sufferings that are inseparable from the disease. She urged nurses to take control of the essentials of nursing, the proper use of fresh air, light, warmth, cleanliness, quiet, and the proper selection and administration of diet, and of all that makes nursing possible.

The adaptation model of nursing assumes the universal importance of promoting adaptation in states of health and disease. The theme of nursing's impact on the adaptation of individuals and groups in society has been repeatedly spelled out in my writings and speeches. No amount of medical knowledge will lessen the accountability for nurses to do what nurses do, that is, manage the environment to promote positive life processes. This might be considered an updating of Nightingale's plea to nurses and it includes the nurse's use of self in the caring interpersonal relationship. I was introduced to this notion in my first nursing textbook, *Interpersonal Relations in Nursing,* by Hildegard Peplau. We no longer had Nightingale lamp-lighting ceremonies, but the connection of my readings and later writings to the "lady with the lamp" attending soldiers in the Crimea was clear to me. One of the joys of the implementation projects on the Roy Adaptation Model has been seeing the professional growth and pride when nurses see more clearly what nursing is, and what it is not.

Nightingale placed the challenge of professional nursing to a society much in need of nursing care. Poverty, poor housing, and a displaced labor force all militated against the "laws of health" taking their natural course. Strange as it may seem, we understand more about these laws today and can even predict health problems from our knowledge of the environment, internal and external. Still we do not fashion an environment in which human life processes can flourish. As Annie Goodrich noted in the forward of an earlier printing of this volume, "It is a tragic fact that, despite almost phenomenal advances in the art and science of living, ignorance, poverty and disease still obtain in great degree." Nurses, then, hear the same plea today to shape the policies that have an impact on people receiving the essentials for health. The Roy Adaptation Model expresses this in terms of peoples' interdependence in a larger social system. Nursing is then called on to enhance positive processes for both individual adaptive systems and macroadaptive systems, to promote health within the society.

DOING THE POSSIBLE AND HUNGERING FOR MORE.

There is a tone of urgency, and some would say even caustic dogmatism, in Nightingale's words and message. Palmer (1983) instead emphasizes her far-reaching and long-lasting efforts as a reformer and as one of the greatest humanitarians of the 19th century. As noted above, she believed in doing all that was possible to promote health. She did not allow lack of scientific knowledge, inadequate social and health care systems, or medical and military commands daunt her. Professional women nurses were to be given the best knowledge available and the responsibility and authority to use all at their disposal to remedy the health problems of the day. She was particularly horrified at the unnecessarily high infant mortality rate and maintained that this did not argue for more children's hospitals, but rather challenged women as to whether it is "better to learn the piano-forte than to learn the laws which subserve the preservation of offspring" (p. 7).

A well-known example of the simple yet revolutionary doctrine that she spent her life promulgating was Nightingale's first rule of nursing, that is, to keep the air within as pure as the air without. She recommends simplifying the air test that indicated the organic matter of the air. "Just as without the use of a thermometer no nurse should ever put a patient into a bath, so should no nurse, or mother, or superintendent be without the air test in any ward, nursery, or sleeping-room" (p. 10). It was clear to her that this meant the development of a simple, self-registering instrument. Such technology was to be taken as far as necessary for nurses to make what she understood as nursing possible. She argued that often it was bad sanitary, bad architectural, and bad administrative arrangements that made it impossible to nurse, therefore nursing should have control over these arrangements.

Sidney Herbert, Secretary at War in the British Cabinet, spoke of Nightingale's appointment to the office of "Superintendent of the female nursing establishment in the English General Military Hospitals in Turkey" as an experiment. Furthermore,

he noted that in this experiment Nightingale's personal qualities, knowledge, power of administration, rank, and position in
society gave her advantages that others did not possess (Palmer,
1983). She did not stop with the challenges she faced in Crimea,
rather, she pushed her reform efforts to include the health of the
nation. Nightingale used her military appointment to argue that
a way of preventing illness in the British soldier was to improve
the health of the nation. Furthermore, nursing was a significant
way to improve the health of the British population. Her premise
was that "... Nature ([God] did not) intend mothers to be always
accompanied by doctors" (p. 7), therefore she declared that the
health of the country was dependent on womankind, that women
should be instructed in the art of health, and that the person to
best accomplish this instruction was the nurse. This thinking
was clearly contrary to the prevailing role given to women in Victorian England.

If Nightingale looked at some of our 20th or 21st century
facts, I wonder what she would do? Around the globe rapid
change in all spheres of human existence—social, political, economic, moral, technologic, environmental, and the like, especially the development and use of information and energy—is
straining the fabric of society. The effect is immeasurably beyond
the turmoil of the Industrial Revolution, when machines took the
place of hand-held tools. Just a few examples from publications I
receive:

Over 60% of Peru's population lives in critical poverty with an
average income of $15.50 per month;
The number of United States residents living in poverty increased by 2.1 million in 1990;
In San Francisco, one in every eight people lives in poverty, even
when the definition of poverty has changed so that a family of
four with an annual income of $13,360 is no longer considered
poor;
The biggest killers in our culture are legal and media-driven,
that is, there are more tobacco- and alcohol-related deaths
each day than deaths from heroin, crack, fire, car accidents,
homicides, and AIDS combined;
Television promotes addiction by passive viewing, producing a
range of emotions from an unreal world without true interactions;
A $150 million, high-tech, maximum security prison is planned
in Colorado designed to allow one guard to control the movements of prisoners in several cell blocks by way of electronic
doors, cameras, and audio equipment, thus eliminating even
minimal contact with other human beings;
One year after Operation Desert Shield/Desert Storm, Iraq's
electric generating capacity and water were restored to only

25% of prewar levels and 300,000 people, mostly children under five years of age, are expected to die from famine and
spreading illness;

The average miles per gallon of gas for cars driven in the United
States is 19, whereas the most fuel-efficient cars developed
run at 121 miles per gallon;

It costs $100 million to build a mile of urban highway and $15
million to build a mile of light rail transit;

Half of all Asian/Pacific Islanders and Native Americans live in
communities with uncontrolled toxic waste;

A United States Senate bill addresses issues of violence against
women, including rape, domestic violence, and crimes against
women on college campuses, for which the medical costs total
over $100 million per year and the human costs are incalcula-
ble;

On any given night, there are approximately 500,00 homeless
people in the United States, and nearly 40% of the total
homeless population in the United States is women and children;

And on and on, until possibly I can amass in a week more evidence of human pain and suffering than Nightingale perceived in her lifetime.

Nightingale would be sure to respond in her characteristic
way, noting that she need not wait until she fully understood
these phenomena, nor definitively prove that a given approach
could relieve such suffering, but rather she would use everything
at her disposal, and all that she could garner from others, to relieve such suffering and find ways to prevent it. She would organize and teach nurses to work with people around the world to
create life-giving environments, to free human bodies and spirits
from all that hinders full life potential. My own commitment in
the late 20th century is even more compelling—to create broad
social reform and to call women, especially nurses, to transform
our world to preserve and promote the well-being of humankind.

This commitment comes directly from who I am and my life
experiences and choices. My family from my father's side is
traced to two brothers who planned to flee the French Revolution
in the 18th century, with one arriving in eastern Canada. From
this branch came the French Canadian General Baureguard,
who is reported to have ordered the first shot of the American
Civil War on Fort Sumter, the stronghold of Union army supplies on an island outside of Charleston. My mother's heritage is
linked to the migrations from England to New England in the
17th century. The early settlers learned to survive from the Native Americans and later flourished as landholders and educators. It is recorded that a Hemenway was injured on the bridge
at Concord, in the battle that marks the opening of the American

Revolution. It is likely that he recovered, since it seems that this same person reappears in a number of battles led by General George Washington. Both of my parents were nourished in a deep religious faith. They raised their large family trusting in Providence, without the economic securities of post-World War suburbia. While working as a pantry girl, then as a maid, in a large urban hospital, my coworkers were Hungarian immigrants, an older woman who fled Russia when the Czar fell, several people with various disabilities, and people of the major ethnic groups of the growing city of Los Angeles, including Chicanos, Blacks, Philippinos, Chinese, and Japanese. At 14 life came to me on a broad scale, and even though I may have been on a different social scale from Nightingale, I feel my particular experience also prepared me to be socially sensitive and concerned.

My religious convictions and commitments somehow made me believe that I could do something to make a difference. The congregation of religious women to which I belong, the Sisters of St. Joseph of Carondelet, was begun by six young women in about 1650 in France who, under the pastoral care of a spiritual director and the Bishop of LePuy, formed a way of religious life contrary to that allowed to women in that day. Rather than maintaining a strict cloister away from the world, they were dedicated to "the practice of all the spiritual and corporal works of mercy of which woman is capable and which will most benefit the ...dear neighbor" (Primitive Constitutions). In practice, these women divided the city into four sectors and went out in pairs to meet the needs in each area. They cared for orphans, the sick poor, young women, prisoners, the destitute, and others in need. They did not shy away from any demands of this new way of life, and like Nightingale, managed to follow their convictions in spite of established limited roles for women. Later in America, my Sisters were caring for soldiers on the fields of the Civil War; they were with frightened families at Pearl Harbor; their homes provided safe harbor for service men and women coming and going to the war in the Pacific; and today they are with suffering people in terrorist-ravaged, economically devastated, and cholera-plagued countries such as Peru.

Community experiences of my young adult, early professional years were filled with strong, selfless women, always in positions of authority—administrator of a hospital, president of a college, or an elected representative to the state legislature. It was only later, with the Women's Movement, that I realized that gender roles in society were not structured as I knew them. I had long taken for granted as a way of life the leadership role of women in all sectors of response to human need, but learned that society was only beginning to provide these experiences for women. The externals of religious life began to change in the 1960s and 1970s, but the convictions reached deeper to bring the "spirit of the founders," seeking "the more" in service to the current needs of people in the changing society. I became part of a core group of Sisters that studied social justice concerns and planned related activities, such as marching with Cesar Chavez as he struggled to bring drinking water and safe toilet facilities to the open fields where the farm workers of California bent their backs and bare hands to the task of picking half the fruit eaten throughout the United States. Our group planned both educational and action-oriented programs for awareness of and involvement in the peace movement and for political and community organization to improve housing, health care, and social services for the poor and homeless. We involved our Sisters and all those who would join us. Throughout the world today, we share the feeling that where one of us is, there we all are, doing all that a woman is capable of for the benefit of her neighbor.

CONCLUSION.

My work as a nurse theorist is my way of looking over the people in the complex environments of the cities (and towns, villages, rural areas, mountains, seas, forests, and space stations) of the next century and joining forces with other women, especially nurses, to bring the best that I know and that I am to provide a perspective to enhance vigor for life, belief in being able to effect change, and a vision of the ideal within the real. If Nightingale could somehow come "back to the future" of the new 21st century, I would simply show her around a bit, then ask where she wants to start with the professional nursing responsibilities facing this generation.

REFERENCES.

Nightingale, F. (1859). *Notes on nursing: What it is, and what it is not.* London: Harrison & Sons.

Palmer, I. (1983). From whence we came. In N. Chaska (Ed.), *The nursing profession: A time to speak* (pp. 3–28). New York: McGraw Hill.

NIGHTINGALE:
THE ENDURING SYMBOL.

Margretta Madden Styles

Florence Nightingale died 20 years before I was born, yet I have been enamored with her as long as I can remember. It's not because I have the need for a hero. It is that nursing has the need for enduring symbols.

ON SYMBOLS.

Symbols carry the message of our essence.

Symbols transmit the culture, the ideals, the mission, and the hopes, expectations, and promises of a profession to its members and to the world at large.

Symbols bind us to one another and to past and future generations of nurses.

They give us our identity.

They remind us of our constant purpose and values.

They rally us to our cause in times of special need.

Symbols, in the form of **words, names, pictures,** or **objects,** are a means of high-speed, high-impact communication. They signal immediately—and almost subliminally—that we are what we are. Through symbols a complex of traditions, beliefs, and acts are conveyed in an instant with exquisite simplicity and clarity.

Enduring symbols are not static. They grow in importance and meaning. They begin as an event that grips us and becomes

---

Margretta Madden Styles, Ed.D., R.N., F.A.A.N., is Livingston Professor of Nursing, University of California, San Francisco, San Francisco, California.

embroidered, and enlarged, and emboldened with passing circumstances and sometimes through nurturance or calculation.

Symbols don't have to be loved by all, nor need they be profound or complete representations. They just have to be recognized—recognized for projecting universal, unique, positive messages about nursing.

Professions without symbols are vulnerable both within and without. The members have no center, no anchor, and no bond. Society, having no handles with which to grasp the meaning and value of the profession and its services, will devise its own symbols or consider the profession not worth comprehending.

The value of symbolism is understood by wise leaders. They know that the effective use of symbolism is both a mark and a task of leadership. Leaders meticulously select, create, and use symbols to reinforce or transform beliefs, behaviors, and images. And leaders themselves sometimes become symbols.

ON NURSING'S SEARCH FOR SYMBOLS.

In recent decades we have searched for a new identity and a new significance for nursing through a succession of symbols.

The starched, pristine, maidenly uniform and cap were abandoned for the lab coat or blue jeans or business suit.

The modest bandage scissors tucked in the pocket were visually exchanged for the bold stethoscope dangling conveniently (and conspicuously) around the neck.

The lamp was replaced, generations later, by telemetry.

The chart, for some, gave way to the clipboard, which in turn has yielded to the computer.

In our self-portrayal, the hospital receded as the community and the college campus loomed larger.

None of these modern physical symbols belongs to nursing alone.

And words. "High tech–high touch," as we describe ourselves, expresses not only the breadth and demands of practice but an internal tension within each of us and within the body of nursing. "If caring were enough...," the slogan of the media campaign of the 1990s, begs it be understood that nursing is more than hands and feet and emotion.

Our symbols of the late 20th century are not a mirage. They rightfully and accurately reflect changes in nursing and changes in nurses. They also reflect the drive for a cognitive, intellectual, high-status image. They reflect an arduous swim for the mainstream of respectability.

What is lost or submerged in the mainstream are the symbols exclusive to nursing, symbols by which nursing alone can be

identified and with which nurses alone can identify and feel
privileged and special.

A profession on the brink of an identity crisis must search for
its roots and restore, reinstate, and reassert its enduring symbols within a contemporary context.

ON FLORENCE NIGHTINGALE AS SYMBOL.

Florence Nightingale is our enduring symbol. Not all nurses
will accept that gladly. For some she is the ancestor we love to
loathe. She has been scorned on occasion by her own professional
progeny as a crackpot, branded as a despot, even sneered at as a
luetic. This is the venom with which we savage our could-be
idols, so that we are left with no peers to look up to.

It is enough that we accept Nightingale for what she was and
is. She was a person with strengths and frailties. She was powerful in her day. She planted the seeds of modern nursing. Her
name survives and, above all others, is universally associated
with nursing, by nurses and the public.

But more important than the fact that she *is* our most enduring symbol is the recognition that she *deserves* to be.

She represents many of the values we continue to hold dear.

The origins of many of today's nursing movements can be
traced to the Nightingale legacy.

We are just coming to grips with some of the dimensions she
ascribed to nursing more that 130 years ago. "...The very elements of nursing are all but unknown," (p. 6) she said then and
may still be muttering to us from the grave.

I am not a historian, not a theoretician, not even much of a
scholar. Perhaps I could call myself a nurse–patriot. But because
of what I am and what I am not, I don't want to be a Nightingale
student, to analyze her every word and deed. Let that be the
work of others. I just want to believe in and draw strength from
my impressions and to let my pride as a nurse take flight on the
wings of fragments of her legend.

- I am staggered by the range of her intellect and interest. The
  same mind conceived and the same hands delivered the soft
  strokes of nursing and the hammer blows of social activism.
  Even today one can feel the bite of her determination.
- I think of her as the original liberated woman and take on new
  self-esteem in knowing that she rejected convention and comfort to clear the path for a calling then alien to the gentry. This
  is a striking personal statement about the importance of our
  work.
- I am proud that so early she brought rationality and theory and
  science—sometimes brilliant, sometimes rudimentary, some-

times mistaken—to clinical practice and health service management, proud that she has been called "the passionate statistician."

• I am amazed at her political cunning, moved by her militancy, and forever inspired by her stirring summons, "No system can endure that does not march."

• I smile that she was preaching vehemently about the environment, the community (or district), sanitation, hygiene, healthy living, and preserving the vitality of patients more than a century before primary health care was elevated to the rank of worldwide gospel at Alma Ata.

I am pleased that other professions too, such as dietetics, various therapies, public health, and hospital management lay claim to her heritage. Yet I know she is truly ours. All of these are "elements of nursing."

These fragments pieced together form a collage of Nightingale as feminist, practitioner, politician, scientist, environmentalist, visionary, reformer—a striking, noble portrait. But I hold still another, a more personal, intimate picture in my mind.

Displayed within a showcase at the entrance to our school is a letter written by Nightingale in 1855 to the parents of a young soldier who died of typhus in the Crimea. She describes his last moments. I fancy that she wrote it late at night fighting to overcome despair and fatigue, after she had finished her rounds with the lamp that, in turn, became her symbol. And I fancy that she wrote similar letters to the loved ones of all of those for whom she cared so deeply and felt so profoundly responsible. And I am moved to tears of pride because I know that nurses everywhere are carrying on the Nightingale tradition in myriad ways and circumstances.

The Nightingale name is ours.
The ideal persists.
The lamp burns on.
The symbol endures.

REFERENCE.

Nightingale, F. (1859). *Notes on nursing: What it is, and what it is not.* London: Harrison & Sons.

NOTES ON NURSING:
STIRRING THE SPIRIT OF REFORM.

John D. Thompson

If one holds that the Civil War was as important to the development of nursing in the United States as the Crimean War was to British nursing, then the publication of *Notes on Nursing* assumes awesome importance. There is much evidence that those concerned with the care of the wounded early in the Civil War were drawing parallels between the British misadventures in the Crimea and the Union experience. This became evident after the First Battle of Bull Run (Manassas), when the retreat of the Union troops turned into a rout and the wounded, exhausted, and sick soldiers crowded into Washington, DC. No hospitals were open to receive them; stores of clean clothing, bandages, and medicine sent by numerous Ladies Aid Associations could not be dispensed to the troops. A quotation from one source, Mary Livermore's *My Story of the War—A Woman's Narrative,* the principle source for documentation of women's involvement in the Civil War, reflected the parallels with Crimea, "All (there) were tied up with official formalism until Florence Nightingale, with her corps of trained nurses and full power to do and command, as well as advise, landed at Scutari, and ordered the store houses opened" (Livermore, 1889, p. 127). Such observations resulted in the founding of the United States Sanitary Commission from the many "Ladies Aid Societies," organizations gathering medical supplies, personal clothing, and medicine for the troops. It was one of history's oddest coincidences that William Russell of the London *Times,* whose reports on the failures at Crimea re-

---

John D. Thompson, R.N., M.S., is Professor Emeritus of Public Health and Nursing Administration, Yale University Schools of Medicine and Nursing, New Haven, Connecticut.

sulted in Nightingale's mission, was an observer at the First Battle of Bull Run. Pressure was put on President Lincoln, who reluctantly gave the approval to establish the Commission, as a "fifth wheel to assist the army."

Bullough and Bullough (1978) point out that *Notes on Nursing* was published in the United States in 1860, one year after its publication in London. There is evidence that the American women who volunteered as nurses read the book. Martin Kaufman (1988), in the *Dictionary of American Nursing Biography,* states that at least two such women read the book before providing nursing care in military hospitals: Louisa May Alcott on the Union side, and Kate Cumming, who established nursing services for the Confederacy.

My own acquaintance with the book began in the place I was trained. It was impossible to ignore Florence Nightingale at Bellevue Hospital in New York. The famous letter recommending the type of nursing school that should be founded at Bellevue was enclosed in a glass "book" and mounted on the wall of the largest classroom. We were frequently reminded of the fact that our school was based on the school at St. Thomas Hospital. It was founded, not so incidentally, by women who were active in the United States Sanitary Commission during the Civil War.

As a nurse and medical administrator trained in public health, I have always been struck by the concern for disease prevention in *Notes on Nursing.* Prevention is the overall theme of the little book, appearing faintly in the first few pages, reinforced throughout the discussion of each element of environmental control necessary to the well-being of the patient. On the second page of text we read, "If a patient is cold, if a patient is feverish, if a patient is faint, if he is sick after taking food, if he has a bed-sore, it is generally the fault not of the disease, but of the nursing" (p. 6).

Toward the end of the book it appears in the undiluted statement of the surgical nurse's duty, "In surgical wards, one duty of every nurse certainly is *prevention....*The surgical nurse must be ever on the watch, ever on her guard, against want of cleanliness, foul air, want of light, and of warmth" (p. 71).

All of this was a very good diagnosis of the type of care at the time. Admission to a hospital or a sick room was too often the first step toward death. Complications such as hospital pyemia or erysipelas were passed from patient to patient. If you weren't deathly ill when you came under treatment, it would not be long before you were. Nightingale was trying to translate her results at Scutari to civilian hospitals and homes. As she stated in *Notes on Hospitals* (1859):

We had during the first seven months of the Crimean campaign a mortality among the troops at the rate of 60 percent per annum

*from disease alone, the rate of mortality which exceeds that of the
great plague in London, and a higher ratio than the mortality in
cholera to the attacks. We had during the last six months of the war
a mortality among our sick not much more than among our healthy
guards at home, and a mortality among our troops in the last five
months two-thirds only of what it is among our troops at home (p.
24).*

The aim of the Commission, which received counsel and advice from Nightingale, was to prevent all disease. They realized
that deaths from wounds were not preventable but that deaths
from disease, malnutrition, and filth were.

Another interesting section of *Notes on Nursing* is the discussion of "Petty Management," although the management turns
out to be anything but petty. Two main aspects of management
are addressed, one on how to ensure that the patient will be well
cared for when the nurse is not there, and another addressing
what it means to be "in charge." The first area treats the subtle
difference between a professional caregiver and a slave. There
are two things the nurse must do: project the probable needs of
the patient, and realize one cannot and should not be with the
patient at all times, although the patient must be informed of
how long the nurse will be absent and what should happen while
she is gone.

One can visualize future generations of charge nurses following the admonition "To be 'in charge' is certainly not only to
carry out the proper measures yourself but to see that everyone
else does so too" (p. 24). Nightingale addresses the problem of
the private duty nurse going into a home and ordering the servants about "under plea of not neglecting the patient" (p. 25).
This is not usually the nurse's fault, she maintains, but the fault
of the person "in charge" of the home.

It is an interesting exercise to contrast the tone and style of
Notes on Nursing with that of *Notes on Hospitals,* written about
the same time. *Notes on Nursing* is much softer in tone, although
still prescriptive, and illustrates its points with anecdotes,
whereas *Notes on Hospitals* is mainly a polemic and is full of statistics, formulas, and facts.

The only table in *Notes on Nursing* is an abstract from the
1851 census reporting on the number, age, and servant status of
nurses in the districts of Great Britain, including Scotland and
Wales. Nightingale comments only mildly on the young ages of
nurses who are domestic servants—over half were under age 20.
These nurses were probably caring for children. One does not get
much of a feel for Nightingale as "passionate statistician" from
Notes on Nursing, which is too bad—that's what she did best!
One must say that Nightingale did not view *Notes on Nursing* as
an instrument of reform—its main purpose was to enlist other

reformers. It is my hope that nursing never loses its passion for reform.

REFERENCES.

Bullough, V.L., & Bullough, B. (1978). *The care of the sick, the emergence of modern nursing.* New York: Prodist.

Kaufman, M. (Ed.). (1988). *Dictionary of American nursing biography.* New York: Greenwood Press.

Livermore, M.A. (1889). *My story of the war—a woman's narrative.* Hartford, CT: A.D. Worthington.

Nightingale, F. (1859). *Notes on hospitals* (1st ed.). London: Longman.

Nightingale, F. (1859). *Notes on nursing: What it is, and what it is not.* London: Harrison & Sons.

NOTES ON NURSING: GUIDELINES FOR CARING THEN AND NOW.

Jean Watson

Would you do nothing then, in cholera, fever...?
—so deep-rooted and universal is the conviction that to give medi-cine is to be doing something, or rather everything; to give air, warmth, cleanliness, &c., is to do nothing....The very elements of...nursing are...little understood (p. 6).

From one century to another, from one turn-of-the-century to another, Florence Nightingale's vision and wisdom ring true and speak to us still. Through the ages her voice can be heard more loudly than ever, if we listen, if we are ready to hear the calling, if we are ready to consider anew her timeless message in this era.

Her century-old thinking about nursing proclaimed and fore-shadowed the emerging caring feminine consciousness still awakening in our time. Nightingale's proclamation was a call to women and to nursing consciousness as the repository of both knowledge and wisdom, a significant social, political, and hu-mane force in overcoming ignorance toward basic health, human caring, and healing.

This health knowledge and wisdom, so desperately needed in her time, remains the call and manifesto of our time—the need to reiterate the interconnection between person and environ-ment, between person and nature, between the inner and outer worlds, between the private and the public, between the physical and the spiritual as part of the natural healing responses of peo-ple and civilizations; the need to systematically develop nursing

---

Jean Watson, R.N., Ph.D., F.A.A.N., is Professor of Nursing, the University of Colorado Health Sciences Center, Boulder, Colorado, and is Director of The Center for Human Caring, Denver, Colorado.

practice; the need to have a developed nursing service where people are cared for by qualified nurses; the need for nurses to not
have to forfeit a proper education; and the need to enhance the
quality of nursing and health services offered to the public.
Even though the roots of nursing throughout time have been
based on a philosophy and commitment to caring and healing,
and all the insights from Nightingale, ironically we find ourselves at the end of the 20th century, a century of revolution in
biomedical science, having to return to the ancient vision of
Nightingale to make a case for basic human caring–healing
health knowledge and practices. Indeed, nursing has never fulfilled the promise of Nightingale.

> ...It is extraordinary that, whereas the laws of the motions of the
> heavenly bodies, far removed as they are from us, are perfectly well
> understood, the laws of the human mind, which are under our ob-
> servation all day and every day, are no better understood than they
> were two thousand years ago. But how much more extraordinary is
> it that...neither mothers...nor nurses of hospitals, are taught any-
> thing about those laws which God has assigned to the relations of
> our bodies with the world in which He has put them (p. 7).

Just as a century ago nursing was considered a "calling,"
there is once again an open call for compassion, commitment, involvement, a passion, if you will, for nurses to recommit to a
"calling" to engage in reform based on basic human caring–healing and health values; reform based on knowledge rooted in ancient feminine wisdom and knowledge, a cosmology of wholeness,
connectedness, and harmony that need to once again be openly
pronounced for personal, public, scientific, and political action.
Nightingales's attunement to the interconnections between
all dimensions of the personal, the public, and the political parallel the voice of contemporary women who remind us again, in
postmodern feminist terms, that the personal is the political.
Thus, the feminist voice of this era takes on deeper significance
when reconsidered within the historical backdrop of Nightingale's strong message to make the private work and world of
women's (caring) knowledge and wisdom a source of public and
political significance. This private, ancient feminine wisdom,
once brought to the public and political consciousness, can become the foundation for societal and system reform, if not transformation.
This ancient Nightingale wisdom is also part of nursing's caring theory. The carative factors in my first caring work are
highly consistent with Nightingale's call for a values-based approach to the nursing profession, oneness of mindbodyspirit with
respect to care needs. We share a concern for the humanistic—
the altruistic, the spiritual, the scientific, the existential, but
also a concern for basic caring practices as well as "the health of

houses." This shared thinking seeks to recognize and restore the connections between person–environment–nature; the connection between physical and metaphysical; the relationship between health and wholeness with respect to such factors as noise, light, air, color, touch, variety of stimuli, and so on.

Caring practices that emerge from my carative factors attend to feelings, relationships, teaching–learning, caring transactions and moments, context, consciousness, and concrete actions related to supportive, protective, or corrective mental, physical, sociocultural and spiritual environment. Variables affecting external and internal environments, such as stress–change, comfort needs, privacy, and clean–aesthetic surroundings, are all carative factors that are very Nightingale in their approach.

This pervasive aspect of nursing, transmitted by Nightingale's writings as well as contemporary caring work, requires that the caring knowledge of women and nurses no longer remain hidden. Nursing's work today again requires strong voices, a being-in-the-world, courageously and convincingly conveying a new proclamation for reform in the personal, public, political, and social thinking and acting of our time.

Caring writing today shares a century-old national and global agenda with Nightingale. We continue to be informed and inspired by the rich, often hidden, ordinary caring–healing knowing of nursing and women. This so-called ordinary knowing Nightingale advocated was also valued as extraordinary. Ordinary knowing becomes extraordinary when we enter into human caring with a spiritual sense of awe and reverence, with a sense of the fantastic. This kind of calling provides us with a clarity of values essential to sustaining compassion, commitment, and caring in instances where people and society are threatened biologically or otherwise. Thus, the ordinary caring taken for granted in nursing transforms into the extraordinary to inform our vision, our way of seeing, our way of being and knowing and doing that Nightingale asserted.

Some of Nightingale's seeing and knowing included ancient insights and values that parallel current human caring theory— theory to once again guide nursing education, praxis, and clinical inquiry that is based on caring as a moral ideal; theory that allows for the spiritual, the transcendent, the whole, while attending to fully embodied being and doing. Some of Nightingale's seeing and knowing included a vision and image of completeness, of beauty and harmony of life, a sense of oneness with all living things.

Some of this timeless Nightingale seeing and knowing is congruent with the emerging caring–healing paradigm of our time that speaks to the natural healing processes, the inner healer, the need for being connected with nature. All of this timeless seeing and knowing presented by Nightingale, a woman of vision, remains. Nevertheless, even though this perspective of seeing and knowing remains and is reflected in contemporary human caring theory in nursing, this so-called extraordinary seeing and knowing is yet to totally emerge in nursing and women's consciousness.

Just as *Notes on Nursing* said that the very elements of nursing are all but unknown, so is this true a century later. One of the messages of nursing caring theory today is a call for the restoration of basic values, commitment, and informed moral action that leads to social and political action. Nursing caring theory continues to reiterate a call for the search for new caring knowledge and caring praxis: practice informed by human values and an ethos of caring. This unknown knowledge requires a continuing search for new relationships between elements of human caring and healing processes and health experiences. Although Nightingale's feminine-based caring–healing model has transcended time and is prophetic for this century's health reform, the model is yet to truly come of age in nursing or the health care system. The enduring Nightingale voice remains before us as part of the pressing public, political, and scientific agendas, in spite of our politically and scientifically renowned turn-of-the-century institutions.

NIGHTINGALE'S ENDURING PUBLIC HEALTH AND HUMAN CARING PROCLAMATIONS.

Is all this premature suffering and death necessary? (p. 7).

If we then reconsider Nightingale in light of a general philosophy and theory of caring her voice parallels the public and political consciousness of today. It is timely to pronounce once again the human significance of basic public health and human caring within the Nightingale model. Today the AIDS epidemic and reports of malaria, measles, and cholera outbreaks around the world match Nightingale's time. Just as in the 1800s, the call today is still a call for reform of basic human caring and health practices with respect to the homeless, the medically indigent, those who are HIV-positive or suffering with AIDS or other incurable or chronic illness—those who are often neglected, such as pregnant women and children.

Calls for health care and system reform are just as worldwide today as they were then. These calls today, which parallel those is Nightingale's time, are in the form of personal, social, and political action. With the blight of the American health care (read sick care) system there are now requests to create "dedicated" caring–healing units and practices in and out of our institutions; calls to deal with the epidemic of diseases caused by social, political, and even scientific neglect; calls to counterbalance the technologic imperatives; calls to attend to basic human comfort measures such as human touch, massage, relaxation, mood change; social and political action calls to attend to the quality of living and dying; calls to encompass natural and aesthetic surroundings that attend to light, form, air, color, and nature; calls to be as equally concerned with and present to the spiritual/metaphysical elements of caring-healing as with the physical; calls to be concerned with relationships and unity and wholeness; calls to be concerned with consciousness and transcendence of self with respect to higher self and one's own inner healer. The contexts for all of these approaches are basic public health issues that are humanitarian as well as scientific and political. Nightingale's earlier thinking calls for a very similar caring—healing model today as part of a mandate for health reform, embedded in caring theory.

POSTMODERN MESSAGES FROM NIGHTINGALE.

Just as at the turn of the past century, we once again need social and political action based on a world view and metaparadgim that has roots in women's wisdom and knowledge. This knowledge can be a basis for a profession, but it is also wisdom beyond knowledge that can be transmitted from woman to woman. The writings of Nightingale remain contemporary and timeless. We can now reconsider the timeless themes, themes that are a part of our awakening, our emerging with our feminine wisdom as part of the social action reform called for as the next century greets us.

In summary, there are several pervasive themes from Nightingale and her time that mirror basic philosophy and theories of human caring in contemporary nursing. They are:

- Restoration of basic nursing caring–healing practices
- Reintegration of the moral, the spiritual, the metaphysical
- Emergence of women's knowledge and values, the feminine spirit
- Return of a "sense of a calling" to the profession
- The public's request for personal and professional caring
- Competencies and commitments
- Honor of the wisdom of connected oneness, wholeness, the interrelationship between and among person–nature–environment/ caring–health–healing
- Recognition of the interrelationship between and among the personal, the political, the social andthe scientific.

Thus, Nightingale's insight and world view hold power and vision for these postmodern times in nursing's history, just as they did in her time. Nightingale's voice still offers prescient recommendations for health care reform that are called for now as loudly as in 1859, when *Notes on Nursing* was written. This reform speaks largely to women and the public about personal health care and health knowledge that everyone must have.

Nightingale's views on nursing, her vision, commitment, and dedication to nursing and nurses continue to be foundational, informative, and inspirational, if not prophetic. Caring–healing— health reform in nursing builds on what we now know as a feminine cosmology, a worldview that Nightingale proclaimed a century ago. This time around nursing can enter the future with authentic connections for both moral and political inspiration and action. Perhaps this time, a century later, postmodern feminist-conscious nursing will finally reclaim its heritage as the health, human caring, and healing profession for the next century.

Are we listening? Do we hear the calling? Are we ready?

REFERENCES.

Pearson, A., Durand, I., & Punton, S. (1987). *Therapeutic nursing: The effect of admission to a nursing unit on patient outcome.* Preliminary report, November. United Kingdom: Oxfordshire Health Authority. Unpublished.

Pearson, A., & McMahon, R. (1991). *Nursing as therapy.* London: Chapman Hall.

Deakin Institute of Nursing Research at Deakin University. (1990–1991). *Annual report.* Victoria, Australia: The Ernestine McKellar Professorial Nursing Unit.

Pembrey, S. (1989). The inaugural lecture: The development of nursing practice—A new contribution. Oxford, UK: Oxford Institute of Nursing.

Nightingale, F. (1859). *Notes on nursing: What it is, and what it is not.* London: Harrison & Sons.

Watson, J. (1979). *Nursing: The philosophy and science of caring.* Boston: Little, Brown.

Watson, J. (1985). *Nursing: Human science and human care.* East Norwalk, CT: Appleton-Century-Crofts.

Watson, J. (1988). Human caring as the moral context for nursing education. *Nursing and Health Care, 9*(8), 422–425.

Watson, J. (1988). New dimensions of human caring theory. *Nursing Science Quarterly, 1*(4), 175–181.

Watson, J. (1990). The moral failure of the patriarchy. *Nursing Outlook, 28*(2), 62–62.

Watson, J. (1990). Caring knowledge and informed moral passion. *Advances in Nursing Science, 13*(1), 15–24.

NOTES ON NURSING:

WHAT IT IS, AND WHAT IT IS NOT.

BY

FLORENCE NIGHTINGALE.

LONDON:

HARRISON, 59, PALL MALL,

BOOKSELLER TO THE QUEEN.

PRINTED BY HARRISON AND SONS,

ST. MARTIN'S LANE, W.C.

ISBN-0-397-54000-0

Facsimile of
the First Edition, printed in London, 1859.
Reproduced by offset in 1946 by
Edward Stern & Company, Inc.,
Philadelphia   Pennsylvania

PREFACE.

THE following notes are by no means intended as a rule of thought by which nurses can teach themselves to nurse, still less as a manual to teach nurses to nurse. They are meant simply to give hints for thought to women who have personal charge of the health of others. Every woman, or at least almost every woman, in England has, at one time or another of her life, charge of the personal health of somebody, whether child or invalid,—in other words, every woman is a nurse. Every day sanitary knowledge, or the knowledge of nursing, or in other words, of how to put the constitution in such a state as that it will have no disease, or that it can recover from disease, takes a higher place. It is recognized as the knowledge which every one ought to have—distinct from medical knowledge, which only a profession can have.

If, then, every woman must, at some time or other of her life, become a nurse, *i.e.*, have charge of somebody's health, how immense and how valuable would be the produce of her united experience if every woman would think how to nurse.

I do not pretend to teach her how, I ask her to teach herself, and for this purpose I venture to give her some hints.

TABLE OF CONTENTS.

NOTES ON NURSING:

WHAT IT IS, AND WHAT IT IS NOT.

SHALL we begin by taking it as a general principle—that all disease, at some period or other of its course, is more or less a reparative process, not necessarily accompanied with suffering: an effort of nature to remedy a process of poisoning or of decay, which has taken place weeks, months, sometimes years beforehand, unnoticed, the termination of the disease being then, while the antecedent process was going on, determined? *Disease a reparative process.*

If we accept this as a general principle we shall be immediately met with anecdotes and instances to prove the contrary. Just so if we were to take, as a principle—all the climates of the earth are meant to be made habitable for man, by the efforts of man—the objection would be immediately raised,—Will the top of Mont Blanc ever be made habitable? Our answer would be, it will be many thousands of years before we have reached the bottom of Mont Blanc in making the earth healthy. Wait till we have reached the bottom before we discuss the top.

In watching disease, both in private houses and in public hospitals, the thing which strikes the experienced observer most forcibly is this, that the symptoms or the sufferings generally considered to be inevitable and incident to the disease are very often not symptoms of the disease at all, but of something quite different—of the want of fresh air, or of light, or of warmth, or of quiet, or of cleanliness, or of punctuality and care in the administration of diet, of each or of all of these. And this quite as much in private as in hospital nursing. *Of the sufferings of disease, always the cause.*

The reparative process which Nature has instituted and which we call disease has been hindered by some want of knowledge or attention, in one or in all of these things, and pain, suffering, or interruption of the whole process sets in.

If a patient is cold, if a patient is feverish, if a patient is faint, if he is sick after taking food, if he has a bed-sore, it is generally the fault not of the disease, but of the nursing.

What nursing ought to do.

I use the word nursing for want of a better. It has been limited to signify little more than the administration of medicines and the application of poultices. It ought to signify the proper use of fresh air, light, warmth, cleanliness, quiet, and the proper selection and administration of diet—all at the least expense of vital power to the patient.

Nursing the sick little understood.

It has been said and written scores of times, that every woman makes a good nurse. I believe, on the contrary, that the very elements of nursing are all but unknown.

By this I do not mean that the nurse is always to blame. Bad sanitary, bad architectural, and bad administrative arrangements often make it impossible to nurse. But the art of nursing ought to include such arrangements as alone make what I understand by nursing, possible.

The art of nursing, as now practised, seems to be expressly constituted to unmake what God had made disease to be, viz., a reparative process.

Nursing ought to assist the reparative process.

To recur to the first objection. If we are asked, Is such or such a disease a reparative process? Can such an illness be unaccompanied with suffering? Will any care prevent such a patient from suffering this or that?—I humbly say, I do not know. But when you have done away with all that pain and suffering, which in patients are the symptoms not of their disease, but of the absence of one or all of the above-mentioned essentials to the success of Nature's reparative processes, we shall then know what are the symptoms of and the sufferings inseparable from the disease.

Another and the commonest exclamation which will be instantly made is—Would you do nothing, then, in cholera, fever, &c.?—so deep-rooted and universal is the conviction that to give medicine is to be doing something, or rather everything; to give air, warmth, cleanliness, &c., is to do nothing. The reply is, that in these and many other similar diseases the exact value of particular remedies and modes of treatment is by no means ascertained, while there is universal experience as to the extreme importance of careful nursing in determining the issue of the disease.

Nursing the well

II. The very elements of what constitutes good nursing are as little understood for the well as for the sick. The same laws of health or of nursing, for they are in reality the same, obtain among the well as among the sick. The breaking of them produces only a less violent consequence among the former than among the latter,—and this sometimes, not always.

It is constantly objected,—"But how can I obtain this medical knowledge? I am not a doctor. I must leave this to doctors."

Little understood.

Oh, mothers of families! You who say this, do you know that one in every seven infants in this civilized land of England perishes before it is one year old? That, in London, two in every five die before they are five years old? And, in the other great cities of

England, nearly one out of two?* "The life duration of tender babies" (as some Saturn, turned analytical chemist, says) "is the most delicate test" of sanitary conditions. Is all this premature suffering and death necessary? Or did Nature intend mothers to be always accompanied by doctors? Or is it better to learn the piano-forte than to learn the laws which subserve the preservation of offspring?

Macaulay somewhere says, that it is extraordinary that, whereas the laws of the motions of the heavenly bodies, far removed as they are from us, are perfectly well understood, the laws of the human mind, which are under our observation all day and every day, are no better understood than they were two thousand years ago.

But how much more extraordinary is it that, whereas what we might call the coxcombries of education—e. g., the elements of astronomy—are now taught to every school-girl, neither mothers of families of any class, nor school-mistresses of any class, nor nurses of children, nor nurses of hospitals, are taught anything about those laws which God has assigned to the relations of our bodies with the world in which He has put them. In other words, the laws which make these bodies, into which He has put our minds, healthy or unhealthy organs of those minds, are all but unlearnt. Not but that these laws—the laws of life—are in a certain measure understood, but not even mothers think it worth their while to study them—to study how to give their children healthy existences. They call it medical or physiological knowledge, fit only for doctors.

Another objection.

We are constantly told,—"But the circumstances which govern our children's healths are beyond our control. What can we do with winds? There is the east wind. Most people can tell before they get up in the morning whether the wind is in the east."

* Upon this fact the most wonderful deductions have been strung. For a long time an announcement something like the following has been going the round of the papers:—"More than 25,000 children die every year in London under 10 years of age; therefore we want a Children's Hospital." This spring there was a prospectus issued, and divers other means taken to this effect:— "There is a great want of sanitary knowledge in women; therefore we want a Women's Hospital." Now, both the above facts are·too sadly true. But what is the deduction? The causes of the enormous child mortality are perfectly well known; they are chiefly want of cleanliness, want of ventilation, want of whitewashing; in one word, defective *household* hygiene. The remedies are just as well known; and among them is certainly not the establishment of a Child's Hospital. This may be a want; just as there may be a want of hospital room for adults. But the Registrar-General would certainly never think of giving us as a cause for the high rate of child mortality in (say) Liverpool that there was not sufficient hospital room for children; nor would he urge upon us, as a remedy, to found a hospital for them.

Again, women, and the best women, are wofully deficient in sanitary knowledge; although it is to women that we must look, first and last, for its application, as far as *household* hygiene is concerned. But who would ever think of citing the institution of a Women's Hospital as the way to cure this want?

We have it, indeed, upon very high authority that there is some fear lest hospitals, as they have been *hitherto*, may not have generally increased, rather than diminished, the rate of mortality—especially of child mortality.

Curious deductions from an excessive death rate.

To this one can answer with more certainty than to the former objections. Who is it who knows when the wind is in the east? Not the Highland drover, certainly, exposed to the east wind, but the young lady who is worn out with the want of exposure to fresh air, to sunlight, &c. Put the latter under as good sanitary circumstances as the former, and she too will not know when the wind is in the east.

I. VENTILATION AND WARMING.

First rule of nursing, to keep the air within as pure as the air without. The very first canon of nursing, the first and the last thing upon which a nurse's attention must be fixed, the first essential to the patient, without which all the rest you can do for him is as nothing, with which I had almost said you may leave all the rest alone, is this: TO KEEP THE AIR HE BREATHES AS PURE AS THE EXTERNAL AIR, WITHOUT CHILLING HIM. Yet what is so little attended to? Even where it is thought of at all, the most extraordinary misconceptions reign about it. Even in admitting air into the patient's room or ward, few people ever think, where that air comes from. It may come from a corridor into which other wards are ventilated, from a hall, always unaired, always full of the fumes of gas, dinner, of various kinds of mustiness; from an underground kitchen, sink, washhouse, water-closet, or even, as I myself have had sorrowful experience, from open sewers loaded with filth; and with this the patient's room or ward is aired, as it is called—poisoned, it should rather be said. Always air from the air without, and that, too, through those windows, through which the air comes freshest. From a closed court, especially if the wind do not blow that way, air may come as stagnant as any from a hall or corridor.

Again, a thing I have often seen both in private houses and institutions. A room remains uninhabited; the fire place is carefully fastened up with a board; the windows are never opened; probably the shutters are kept always shut; perhaps some kind of stores are kept in the room; no breath of fresh air can by possibility enter into that room, nor any ray of sun. The air is as stagnant, musty, and corrupt as it can by possibility be made. It is quite ripe to breed small-pox, scarlet fever, diphtheria, or anything else you please.*

Yet the nursery, ward, or sick room adjoining will positively be aired (?) by having the door opened into that room. Or children will be put into that room, without previous preparation, to sleep.

A short time ago a man walked into a back-kitchen in Queen

Why are uninhabited rooms shut up?   * The common idea as to uninhabited rooms is, that they may safely be left with doors, windows, shutters, and chimney board, all closed—hermetically sealed if possible—to keep out the dust, it is said; and that no harm will happen if the room is but opened a short hour before the inmates are put in. I have often been asked the question for uninhabited rooms—But when ought the windows to be opened? The answer is—When ought they to be shut?

square, and cut the throat of a poor consumptive creature, sitting by the fire. The murderer did not deny the act, but simply said, "It's all right." Of course he was mad.

But in our case, the extraordinary thing is that the victim says, "It's all right," and that we are not mad. Yet, although we "nose" the murderers, in the musty unaired unsunned room, the scarlet fever which is behind the door, or the fever and hospital gangrene which are stalking among the crowded beds of a hospital ward, we say, "It's all right."

With a proper supply of windows, and a proper supply of fuel *Without chill.* in open fire places, fresh air is comparatively easy to secure when your patient or patients are in bed. Never be afraid of open windows then. People don't catch cold in bed. This is a popular fallacy. With proper bed-clothes and hot bottles, if necessary, you can always keep a patient warm in bed, and well ventilate him at the same time.

But a careless nurse, be her rank and education what it may, will stop up every cranny and keep a hot-house heat when her patient is in bed,—and, if he is able to get up, leave him comparatively unprotected. The time when people take cold (and there are many ways of taking cold, besides a cold in the nose,) is when they first get up after the two-fold exhaustion of dressing and of having had the skin relaxed by many hours, perhaps days, in bed, and thereby rendered more incapable of re-action. Then the same temperature which refreshes the patient in bed may destroy the patient just risen. And common sense will point out that, while purity of air is essential, a temperature must be secured which shall not chill the patient. Otherwise the best that can be expected will be a feverish re-action.

To have the air within as pure as the air without, it is not necessary, as often appears to be thought, to make it as cold.

In the afternoon again, without care, the patient whose vital powers have then risen often finds the room as close and oppressive as he found it cold in the morning. Yet the nurse will be terrified, if a window is opened*.

I know an intelligent humane house surgeon who makes a *Open windows.* practice of keeping the ward windows open. The physicians and surgeons invariably close them while going their rounds; and the house surgeon very properly as invariably opens them whenever the doctors have turned their backs.

In a little book on nursing, published a short time ago, we are told, that "with proper care it is very seldom that the windows cannot be opened for a few minutes twice in the day to admit fresh

---

* It is very desirable that the windows in a sick room should be such as that the patient shall, if he can move about, be able to open and shut them easily himself. In fact the sick room is very seldom kept aired if this is not the case— so very few people have any perception of what is a healthy atmosphere for the sick. The sick man often says, "This room where I spend 22 hours out of the 24 is fresher than the other where I only spend 2. Because here I can manage the windows myself." And   is true.

air from without." I should think not; nor twice in the hour either. It only shows how little the subject has been considered.

What kind of warmth desirable. Of all methods of keeping patients warm the very worst certainly is to depend for heat on the breath and bodies of the sick. I have known a medical officer keep his ward windows hermetically closed, thus exposing the sick to all the dangers of an infected atmosphere, because he was afraid that, by admitting fresh air, the temperature of the ward would be too much lowered. This is a destructive fallacy.

To attempt to keep a ward warm at the expense of making the sick repeatedly breathe their own hot, humid, putrescing atmosphere is a certain way to delay recovery or to destroy life.

Bedrooms almost universally foul. Do you ever go into the bed-rooms of any persons of any class, whether they contain one, two, or twenty people, whether they hold sick or well, at night, or before the windows are opened in the morning, and ever find the air anything but unwholesomely close and foul? And why should it be so? And of how much importance it is that it should not be so? During sleep, the human body, even when in health, is far more injured by the influence of foul air than when awake. Why can't you keep the air all night, then, as pure as the air without in the rooms you sleep in? But for this, you must have sufficient outlet for the impure air you make yourselves to go out; sufficient inlet for the pure air from without to come in. You must have open chimneys, open windows, or ventilators; no close curtains round your beds; no shutters or curtains to your windows, none of the contrivances by which you undermine your own health or destroy the chances of recovery of your sick.*

An air-test of essential consequence. * Dr. Angus Smith's air test, if it could be made of simpler application, would be invaluable to use in every sleeping and sick room. Just as without the use of a thermometer no nurse should ever put a patient into a bath, so should no nurse, or mother, or superintendent be without the air test in any ward, nursery, or sleeping-room. If the main function of a nurse is to maintain the air within the room as fresh as the air without, without lowering the temperature, then she should always be provided with a thermometer which indicates the temperature, with an air test which indicates the organic matter of the air. But to be used, the latter must be made as simple a little instrument as the former, and both should be self-registering. The senses of nurses and mothers become so dulled to foul air that they are perfectly unconscious of what an atmosphere they have let their children, patients, or charges, sleep in. But if the tell-tale air-test were to exhibit in the morning, both to nurses and patients and to the superior officer going round, what the atmosphere has been during the night, I question if any greater security could be afforded against a recurrence of the misdemeanour.

And oh; the crowded national school! where so many children's epidemics have their origin, what a tale its air-test would tell! We should have parents saying, and saying rightly, "I will not send my child to that school, the air-test stands at 'Horrid.'" And the dormitories of our great boarding schools! Scarlet fever would be no more ascribed to contagion, but to its right cause, the air-test standing at "Foul."

We should hear no longer of "Mysterious Dispensations," and of "Plague and Pestilence," being "in God's hands," when, so far as we know, He has put them into our own. The little air-test would both betray the cause of these "mysterious pestilences," and call upon us to remedy it.

A careful nurse will keep a constant watch over her sick, especially weak, protracted, and collapsed cases, to guard against the effects of the loss of vital heat by the patient himself. In certain diseased states much less heat is produced than in health ; and there is a constant tendency to the decline and ultimate extinction of the vital powers by the call made upon them to sustain the heat of the body. Cases where this occurs should be watched with the greatest care from hour to hour, I had almost said from minute to minute. The feet and legs should be examined by the hand from time to time, and whenever a tendency to chilling is discovered, hot bottles, hot bricks, or warm flannels, with some warm drink, should be made use of until the temperature is restored. The fire should be, if necessary, replenished. Patients are frequently lost in the latter stages of disease from want of attention to such simple precautions. The nurse may be trusting to the patient's diet, or to his medicine, or to the occasional dose of stimulant which she is directed to give him, while the patient is all the while sinking from want of a little external warmth. Such cases happen at all times, even during the height of summer. This fatal chill is most apt to occur towards early morning at the period of the lowest temperature of the twenty-four hours, and at the time when the effect of the preceding day's diets is exhausted. *[marginal note:* When warmth must be most carefully looked to.*]*

Generally speaking, you may expect that weak patients will suffer cold much more in the morning than in the evening. The vital powers are much lower. If they are feverish at night, with burning hands and feet, they are almost sure to be chilly and shivering in the morning. But nurses are very fond of heating the foot-warmer at night, and of neglecting it in the morning, when they are busy. I should reverse the matter.

All these things require common sense and care. Yet perhaps in no one single thing is so little common sense shewn, in all ranks, as in nursing.*

The extraordinary confusion between cold and ventilation, in the minds of even well educated people, illustrates this. To make a room cold is by no means necessarily to ventilate it. Nor is it at all necessary, in order to ventilate a room, to chill it. Yet, if a nurse finds a room close, she will let out the fire, thereby making it closer, or she will open the door into a cold room, without a fire, or an open window in it, by way of improving the ventilation. *[marginal note:* Cold air not ventilation, nor fresh air a method of chill.*]*

---

* With private sick, I think, but certainly with hospital sick, the nurse should never be satisfied as to the freshness of their atmosphere, unless she can feel the air gently moving over her face, when still.

But it is often observed that nurses who make the greatest outcry against open windows are those who take the least pains to prevent dangerous draughts. The door of the patients' room or ward *must* sometimes stand open to allow of persons passing in and out, or heavy things being carried in and out. The careful nurse will keep the door shut while she shuts the windows, and then, and not before, set the door open, so that a patient may not be left sitting up in bed, perhaps in a profuse perspiration, directly in the draught between the open door and window. Neither, of course, should a patient, while being washed or in any way exposed, remain in the draught of an open window or door.

The safest atmosphere of all for a patient is a good fire and an open window, excepting in extremes of temperature. (Yet no nurse can ever be made to understand this.) To ventilate a small room without draughts of course requires more care than to ventilate a large one.

Night air.

Another extraordinary fallacy is the dread of night air. What air can we breathe at night but night air? The choice is between pure night air from without and foul night air from within. Most people prefer the latter. An unaccountable choice. What will they say if it is proved to be true that fully one-half of all the disease we suffer from is occasioned by people sleeping with their windows shut? An open window most nights in the year can never hurt any one. This is not to say that light is not necessary for recovery. In great cities, night air is often the best and purest air to be had in the twenty-four hours. I could better understand in towns shutting the windows during the day than during the night, for the sake of the sick. The absence of smoke, the quiet, all tend to making night the best time for airing the patients. One of our highest medical authorities on Consumption and Climate has told me that the air in London is never so good as after ten o'clock at night.

Air from the outside. Open your windows, shut your doors.

Always air your room, then, from the outside air, if possible. Windows are made to open; doors are made to shut—a truth which seems extremely difficult of apprehension. I have seen a careful nurse airing her patient's room through the door, near to which were two gaslights, (each of which consumes as much air as eleven men), a kitchen, a corridor, the composition of the atmosphere in which consisted of gas, paint, foul air, never changed, full of effluvia, including a current of sewer air from an ill-placed sink, ascending in a continual stream by a well-staircase, and discharging themselves constantly into the patient's room. The window of the said room, if opened, was all that was desirable to air it. Every room must be aired from without—every passage from without. But the fewer passages there are in a hospital the better.

Smoke.

If we are to preserve the air within as pure as the air without, it is needless to say that the chimney must not smoke. Almost all smoky chimneys can be cured—from the bottom, not from the top. Often it is only necessary to have an inlet for air to supply the fire, which is feeding itself, for want of this, from its own chimney. On the other hand, almost all chimneys can be made to smoke by a careless nurse, who lets the fire get low and then overwhelms it with coal; not, as we verily believe, in order to spare herself trouble, (for very rare is unkindness to the sick), but from not thinking what she is about.

Airing damp things in a patient's room.

In laying down the principle that the first object of the nurse must be to keep the air breathed by her patient as pure as the air without, it must not be forgotten that everything in the room which can give off effluvia, besides the patient, evaporates itself into his air. And it follows that there ought to be nothing in the room, excepting him, which can give off effluvia or moisture. Out of all damp towels, &c., which become dry in the room, the damp, of course, goes into the patient's air. Yet this "of course" seems as little thought of, as if it were an obsolete fiction. How very seldom you see a nurse who acknowledges by her practice that nothing at all ought to be aired in the patient's room, that nothing at all ought to be cooked at the patient's fire! Indeed the arrangements often make this rule impossible to observe.

If the nurse be a very careful one, she will, when the patient leaves his bed, but not his room, open the sheets wide, and throw the bed clothes back, in order to air his bed. And she will spread the wet towels or flannels carefully out upon a horse, in order to dry them. Now either these bed-clothes and towels are not dried and aired, or they dry and air themselves into the patient's air. And whether the damp and effluvia do him most harm in his air or in his bed, I leave to you to determine, for I cannot.

Even in health people cannot repeatedly breathe air in which **Effluvia from** they live with impunity, on account of its becoming charged with **excreta.** unwholesome matter from the lungs and skin. In disease where everything given off from the body is highly noxious and dangerous, not only must there be plenty of ventilation to carry off the effluvia, but everything which the patient passes must be instantly removed away, as being more noxious than even the emanations from the sick.

Of the fatal effects of the effluvia from the excreta it would seem unnecessary to speak, were they not so constantly neglected. Concealing the utensils behind the vallance to the bed seems all the precaution which is thought necessary for safety in private nursing. Did you but think for one moment of the atmosphere under that bed, the saturation of the under side of the mattress with the warm evaporations, you would be startled and frightened too!

The use of any chamber utensil *without a lid** should be utterly **Chamber uten-** abolished, whether among sick or well. You can easily convince **sils without** yourself of the necessity of this absolute rule, by taking one with a **lids.**

---

* But never, never should the possession of this indispensable lid confirm you **Don't make** in the abominable practice of letting the chamber utensil remain in a patient's **your sick-room** room unemptied, except once in the 24 hours, *i.e.*, when the bed is made. Yes, **into a sewer.** impossible as it may appear, I have known the best and most attentive nurses guilty of this; aye, and have known, too, a patient afflicted with severe diarrhœa for ten days, and the nurse (a very good one) not know of it, because the chamber utensil (one with a lid) was emptied only once in the 24 hours, and that by the housemaid who came in and made the patient's bed every evening. As well might you have a sewer under the room, or think that in a water closet the plug need be pulled up but once a day. Also take care that your *lid*, as well as your utensil, be always thoroughly rinsed.

If a nurse declines to do these kinds of things for her patient, "because it is not her business," I should say that nursing was not her calling. I have seen surgical "sisters," women whose hands were worth to them two or three guineas a-week, down upon their knees scouring a room or hut, because they thought it otherwise not fit for their patients to go into. I am far from wishing nurses to scour. It is a waste of power. But I do say that these women had the true nurse-calling—the good of their sick first, and second only the consideration what it was their "place" to do—and that women who wait for the housemaid to do this, or for the charwoman to do that, when their patients are suffering, have not the *making* of a nurse in them.

lid, and examining the under side of that lid. It will be found always covered, whenever the utensil is not empty, by condensed offensive moisture. Where does that go, when there is no lid?

Earthenware, or if there is any wood, highly polished and varnished wood, are the only materials fit for patients' utensils. The very lid of the old abominable close-stool is enough to breed a pestilence. It becomes saturated with offensive matter, which scouring is only wanted to bring out. I prefer an earthenware lid as being always cleaner. But there are various good new-fashioned arrangements.

Abolish slop-pails. A slop-pail should never be brought into a sick room. It should be a rule invariable, rather more important in the private house than elsewhere, that the utensil should be carried directly to the water-closet, emptied there, rinsed there, and brought back. There should always be water and a cock in every water-closet for rinsing. But even if there is not, you must carry water there to rinse with. I have actually seen, in the private sick room, the utensils emptied into the foot-pan, and put back unrinsed under the bed. I can hardly say which is most abominable, whether to do this or to rinse the utensil *in* the sick room. In the best hospitals it is now a rule that no slop-pail shall ever be brought into the wards, but that the utensils shall be carried direct to be emptied and rinsed at the proper place. I would it were so in the private house.

Fumigations. Let no one ever depend upon fumigations, "disinfectants," and the like, for purifying the air. The offensive thing, not its smell, must be removed. A celebrated medical lecturer began one day "Fumigations, gentlemen, are of essential importance. They make such an abominable smell that they compel you to open the window." I wish all the disinfecting fluids invented made such an "abominable smell" that they forced you to admit fresh air. That would be a useful invention.

II.—HEALTH OF HOUSES. *

Health of houses. Five points essential. There are five essential points in securing the health of houses:—

1. Pure air.
2. Pure water.
3. Efficient drainage.
4. Cleanliness.
5. Light.

Health of carriages. * The health of carriages, especially close carriages, is not of sufficient universal importance to mention here, otherwise than cursorily. Children, who are always the most delicate test of sanitary conditions, generally cannot enter a close carriage without being sick—and very lucky for them that it is so. A close carriage, with the horse-hair cushions and linings always saturated with organic matter, if to this be added the windows up, is one of the most unhealthy of human receptacles. The idea of taking an *airing* in it is something preposterous. Dr. Angus Smith has shown that a crowded railway carriage, which goes at the rate of 30 miles an hour, is as unwholesome as the strong smell of a sewer, or as a back yard in one of the most unhealthy courts off one of the most unhealthy streets in Manchester.

Without these, no house can be healthy.   And it will be unhealthy just in proportion as they are deficient.

1. To have pure air, your house must be so constructed as that the outer atmosphere shall find its way with ease to every corner of it. House architects hardly ever consider this.   The object in building a house is to obtain the largest interest for the money, not to save doctors' bills to the tenants.   But, if tenants should ever become so wise as to refuse to occupy unhealthily constructed houses, and if Insurance Companies should ever come to understand their interest so thoroughly as to pay a Sanitary Surveyor to look after the houses where their clients live, speculative architects would speedily be brought to their senses.   As it is, they build what pays best.   And there are always people foolish enough to take the houses they build. And if in the course of time the families die off, as is so often the case, nobody ever thinks of blaming any but Providence* for the result.   Ill-informed medical men aid in sustaining the delusion, by laying the blame on " current contagions."   Badly constructed houses do for the healthy what badly constructed hospitals do for the sick. Once insure that the air in a house is stagnant, and sickness is certain to follow. *[Pure air.]*

2. Pure water is more generally introduced into houses than it used to be, thanks to the exertions of the sanitary reformers. Within the last few years, a large part of London was in the daily habit of using water polluted by the drainage of its sewers and water closets.   This has happily been remedied.   But, in many parts of the country, well water of a very impure kind is used for domestic purposes.   And when epidemic disease shows itself, persons using such water are almost sure to suffer. *[Pure water.]*

3. It would be curious to ascertain by inspection, how many houses in London are really well drained.   Many people would say, surely all or most of them.   But many people have no idea in what good drainage consists.   They think that a sewer in the street, and a pipe leading to it from the house is good drainage.   All the while the sewer may be nothing but a laboratory from which epidemic disease and ill health is being distilled into the house.   No house with any untrapped drain pipe communicating immediately with a sewer, whether it be from water closet, sink, or gully-grate, can ever be healthy.   An untrapped sink may at any time spread fever or pyæmia among the inmates of a palace. *[Drainage.]*

The ordinary oblong sink is an abomination.   That great surface of stone, which is always left wet, is always exhaling into the air.   I have known whole houses and hospitals smell of the sink.   I have met just as strong a stream of sewer air coming up the back stair-case of a grand London house from the sink, as I have ever met at *[Sinks.]*

* God lays down certain physical laws.   Upon His carrying out such laws depends our responsibility (that much abused word), for how could we have any responsibility for actions, the results of which we could not foresee—which would be the case if the carrying out of His laws were *not* certain.   Yet we seem to be continually expecting that He will work a miracle—*i. e.* break His own laws expressly to relieve us of responsibility.

Scutari; and I have seen the rooms in that house all ventilated by the open doors, and the passages all *un*ventilated by the closed windows, in order that as much of the sewer air as possible might be conducted into and retained in the bed-rooms. It is wonderful. Another great evil in house construction is carrying drains underneath the house. Such drains are never safe. All house drains should begin and end outside the walls. Many people will readily admit, as a theory, the importance of these things. But how few are there who can intelligently trace disease in their households to such causes! Is it not a fact, that when scarlet fever, measles, or small-pox appear among the children, the very first thought which occurs is, "where" the children can have "caught" the disease? And the parents immediately run over in their minds all the families with whom they may have been. They never think of looking at home for the source of the mischief. If a neighbour's child is seized with small pox, the first question which occurs is whether it had been vaccinated. No one would undervalue vaccination; but it becomes of doubtful benefit to society when it leads people to look abroad for the source of evils which exist at home.

Cleanliness. 4. Without cleanliness, within and without your house, ventilation is comparatively useless. In certain foul districts of London, poor people used to object to open their windows and doors because of the foul smells that came in. Rich people like to have their stables and dunghill near their houses. But does it ever occur to them that with many arrangements of this kind it would be safer to keep the windows shut than open? You cannot have the air of the house pure with dung heaps under the windows. These are common all over London. And yet people are surprised that their children, brought up in large "well-aired" nurseries and bed-rooms suffer from children's epidemics. If they studied Nature's laws in the matter of children's health, they would not be so surprised.

There are other ways of having filth inside a house besides having dirt in heaps. Old papered walls of years' standing, dirty carpets, uncleansed furniture, are just as ready sources of impurity to the air as if there were a dung-heap in the basement. People are so unaccustomed from education and habits to consider how to make a home healthy, that they either never think of it at all, and take every disease as a matter of course, to be "resigned to" when it comes "as from the hand of Providence;" or if they ever entertain the idea of preserving the health of their household as a duty, they are very apt to commit all kinds of "negligences and ignorances" in performing it.

Light. 5. A dark house is always an unhealthy house, always an ill-aired house, always a dirty house. Want of light stops growth, and promotes scrofula, rickets, &c., among the children.

People lose their health in a dark house, and if they get ill they cannot get well again in it. More will be said about this farther on.

Three common errors in managing the health of houses. Three out of many "negligences and ignorances" in managing the health of houses generally, I will here mention as specimens—1. That the female head in charge of any building does not think it necessary to visit every hole and corner of it every day. How can she expect those who are under 'her to be more careful to maintain her house in a healthy condition than she who is in charge of it?—2. That it is not considered essential to air, to sun, and to clean rooms while uninhabited; which is simply ignoring the first elementary notion of sanitary things, and laying the ground ready for all kinds of diseases.—3. That the window, and one window, is considered enough to air a room. Have you never observed that any room without a fire-place is always close? And, if you have a fire-place, would you cram it up not only with a chimney-board, but perhaps with a great wisp of brown paper, in the throat of the chimney— to prevent the soot from coming down, you say? If your chimney is foul, sweep it; but don't expect that you can ever air a room with only one aperture; don't suppose that to shut up a room is the way to keep it clean. It is the best way to foul the room and all that is in it. Don't imagine that if you, who are in charge, don't look to all these things yourself, those under you will be more careful than you are. It appears as if the part of a mistress now is to complain of her servants, and to accept their excuses—not to show them how there need be neither complaints made nor excuses.

But again, to look to all these things yourself does not mean to do them yourself. "I always open the windows," the head in charge often says. If you do it, it is by so much the better, certainly, than if it were not done at all. But can you not insure that it is done when not done by yourself? Can you insure that it is not undone when your back is turned? This is what being "in charge" means. And a very important meaning it is, too. The former only implies that just what you can do with your own hands is done. The latter that what ought to be done is always done. Head in charge must see to House Hygiene, not do it herself.

And now, you think these things trifles, or at least exaggerated. But what you "think" or what I "think" matters little. Let us see what God thinks of them. God always justifies His ways. While we are thinking, He has been teaching. I have known cases of hospital pyæmia quite as severe in handsome private houses as in any of the worst hospitals, and from the same cause, viz., foul air. Yet nobody learnt the lesson. Nobody learnt *anything* at all from it. They went on *thinking*—thinking that the sufferer had scratched his thumb, or that it was singular that "all the servants" had "whitlows," or that something was "much about this year; there is always sickness in our house." This is a favourite mode of thought—leading *not* to inquire what is the uniform cause of these general "whitlows," but to stifle all inquiry. In what sense is "sickness" being "always there," a justification of its being "there" at all? Does God think of these things so seriously?

I will tell you what was the cause of this hospital pyæmia being in that large private house. It was that the sewer air from an ill-placed sink was carefully conducted into all the rooms by sedulously opening all the doors, and closing all the passage windows. It was that the slops were emptied into the foot pans;—it was that the utensils were never properly rinsed;—it was that the chamber How does He carry out His laws?

c

crockery was rinsed with dirty water;—it was that the beds were never properly shaken, aired, picked to pieces, or changed. It was that the carpets and curtains were always musty;—it was that the furniture was always dusty ; it was that the papered walls were saturated with dirt ;—it was that the floors were never cleaned ;—it was that the uninhabited rooms were never sunned, or cleaned, or aired ; —it was that the cupboards were always reservoirs of foul air;—it was that the windows were always tight shut up at night;—it was that no window was ever systematically opened, even in the day, or that the right window was not opened. A person gasping for air might open a window for himself. But the servants were not taught to open the windows, to shut the doors ; or they opened the windows upon a dank well between high walls, not upon the airier court ; or they opened the room doors into the unaired halls and passages, by way of airing the rooms. Now all this is not fancy, but fact.

How does He teach His laws? In that handsome house I have known in one summer three cases of hospital pyæmia, one of phlebitis, two of consumptive cough : all the *immediate* products of foul air. When, in temperate climates, a house is more unhealthy in summer than in winter, it is a certain sign of something wrong. Yet nobody learns the lesson. Yes, God always justifies His ways. He is teaching while you are not learning. This poor body loses his finger, that one loses his life. And all from the most easily preventible causes.*

Physical degeneration in families. Its causes. The houses of the grandmothers and great grandmothers of this generation, at least the country houses, with front door and back door always standing open, winter and summer, and a thorough draught always blowing through—with all the scrubbing, and cleaning, and polishing, and scouring which used to go on, the grandmothers, and still more the great grandmothers, always out of doors and never with a bonnet on except to go to church, these things entirely account for the fact so often seen of a great grandmother, who was a tower of physical vigour descending into a grandmother perhaps a little less vigorous but still sound as a bell and healthy to the core, into a mother languid and confined to her carriage and house, and lastly into a daughter sickly and confined to her bed. For, remember, even with a general decrease of mortality you may often find a race thus degenerating and still oftener a family. You may see poor little feeble washed-out rags, children of a noble stock, suffering morally and physically, throughout their useless, degenerate

Servants' rooms. * I must say a word about servants' bed-rooms. From the way they are built, but oftener from the way they are kept, and from no intelligent inspection whatever being exercised over them, they are almost invariably dens of foul air, and the "servants' health" suffers in an "unaccountable" (?) way, even in the country. For I am by no means speaking only of London houses, where too often servants are put to live under the ground and over the roof. But in a country "*mansion*," which was really a "mansion," (not after the fashion of advertisements), I have known three maids who slept in the same room ill of scarlet fever. "How catching it is," was of course the remark. One look at the room, one smell of the room, was quite enough. It was no longer "unaccountable." The room was not a small one ; it was up stairs, and it had two large windows—but nearly every one of the neglects enumerated above was there.

lives, and yet people who are going to marry and to bring more such into the world, will consult nothing but their own convenience as to where they are to live, or how they are to live.

With regard to the health of houses where there is a sick person, it often happens that the sick room is made a ventilating shaft for the rest of the house. For while the house is kept as close, unaired, and dirty as usual, the window of the sick room is kept a little open always, and the door occasionally. Now, there are certain sacrifices which a house with one sick person in it does make to that sick person: it ties up its knocker; it lays straw before it in the street. Why can't it keep itself thoroughly clean and unusually well aired, in deference to the sick person ? Don't make your sick-room into a ventilating shaft for the whole house.

We must not forget what, in ordinary language, is called "Infection;"*—a thing of which people are generally so afraid that they frequently follow the very practice in regard to it which they ought to avoid. Nothing used to be considered so infectious or contagious as small pox; and people not very long ago used to cover up patients with heavy bed clothes, while they kept up large fires and shut the windows. Small pox, of course, under this *régime*, is very "infectious." People are somewhat wiser now in their management of this disease. They have ventured to cover the patients lightly and to keep the windows open; and we hear much less of the "infection" of small pox than we used to do. But do people in our days act with more wisdom on the subject of "infection" in fevers—scarlet fever, measles, &c.—than their forefathers did with small pox ? Does not the popular idea of "infection" involve that people should take greater care of themselves than of the patient ? that, for instance, it is safer not to be too much with the patient, not to attend too much to his wants ? Perhaps the best illustration of the utter absurdity of this view of duty in attending on "infectious" diseases is afforded by what was very recently the practice, if it is Infection.

* Is it not living in a continual mistake to look upon diseases, as we do now, as separate entities, which *must* exist, like cats and dogs ? instead of looking upon them as conditions, like a dirty and a clean condition, and just as much under our own control ; or rather as the reactions of kindly nature, against the conditions in which we have placed ourselves. Diseases are not individuals arranged in classes, like cats and dogs, but conditions growing out of one another.

I was brought up, both by scientific men and ignorant women, distinctly to believe that small-pox, for instance, was a thing of which there was once a first specimen in the world, which went on propagating itself, in a.perpetual chain of descent, just as much that there was a first dog, (or a first pair of dogs), and that small-pox would not begin itself any more than a new dog would begin without there having been a parent dog.

Since then I have seen with my eyes and smelt with my nose small-pox growing up in first specimens, either in close rooms or in overcrowded wards, where it could not by any possibility have been " caught," but must have begun.

Nay, more, I have seen diseases begin, grow up, and pass into one another. Now, dogs do not pass into cats.

I have seen, for instance, with a little overcrowding, continued fever grow up ; and with a little more, typhoid fever ; and with a little more, typhus, and all in the same ward or hut.

Would it not be far better, truer, and more practical, if we looked upon disease in this light ?

For diseases, as all experience shows, are adjectives, not noun substantives.

not so even now, in some of the European lazarets—in which the plague-patient used to be condemned to the horrors of filth, over-crowding, and want of ventilation, while the medical attendant was ordered to examine the patient's tongue through an opera-glass and to toss him a lancet to open his abscesses with!

True nursing ignores infection, except to prevent it. Cleanliness and fresh air from open windows, with unremitting attention to the patient, are the only defence a true nurse either asks or needs.

Wise and humane management of the patient is the best safe-guard against infection.

Why must
children have
measles, &c. ? There are not a few popular opinions, in regard to which it is useful at times to ask a question or two. For example, it is com-monly thought that children must have what are commonly called "children's epidemics," "current contagions," &c., in other words, that they are born to have measles, hooping-cough, perhaps even scarlet fever, just as they are born to cut their teeth, if they live.

Now, do tell us, why must a child have measles?

Oh because, you say, we cannot keep it from infection—other children have measles—and it must take them—and it is safer that it should.

But why must other children have measles? And if they have, why must yours have them too?

If you believed in and observed the laws for preserving the health of houses which inculcate cleanliness, ventilation, white-washing, and other means, and which, by the way, *are laws*, as implicitly as you believe in the popular opinion, for it is nothing more than an opinion, that your child must have children's epidemics, don't you think that upon the whole your child would be more likely to escape altogether?

III. PETTY MANAGEMENT.

Petty
management. All the results of good nursing, as detailed in these notes, may be spoiled or utterly negatived by one defect, viz.: in petty manage-ment, or, in other words, by not knowing how to manage that what you do when you are there, shall be done when you are not there. The most devoted friend or nurse cannot be always *there*. Nor is it desirable that she should. And she may give up her health, all her other duties, and yet, for want of a little management, be not one-half so efficient as another who is not one-half so devoted, but who has this art of multiplying herself—that is to say, the patient of the first will not really be so well cared for, as the patient of the second.

It is as impossible in a book to teach a person in charge of sick how to *manage*, as it is to teach her how to nurse. Circumstances must vary with each different case. But it *is* possible to press upon her to think for herself: Now what does happen during my absence? I am obliged to be away on Tuesday. But fresh air, or punctuality is not less important to my patient on Tuesday than it was on

Monday. Or: At 10 P.M. I am never with my patient; but quiet is of no less consequence to him at 10 than it was at 5 minutes to 10.

Curious as it may seem, this very obvious consideration occurs comparatively to few, or, if it does occur, it is only to cause the devoted friend or nurse to be absent fewer hours or fewer minutes from her patient—not to arrange so as that no minute and no hour shall be for her patient without the essentials of her nursing.

A very few instances will be sufficient, not as precepts, but as illustrations. _Illustrations of the want of it._

A strange washerwoman, coming late at night for the "things," will burst in by mistake to the patient's sick-room, after he has fallen into his first doze, giving him a shock, the effects of which are irremediable, though he himself laughs at the cause, and probably never even mentions it. The nurse who is, and is quite right to be, at her supper, has not provided that the washerwoman shall not lose her way and go into the wrong room. _Strangers coming into the sick room._

The patient's room may always have the window open. But the passage outside the patient's room, though provided with several large windows, may never have one open. Because it is not understood that the charge of the sick-room extends to the charge of the passage. And thus, as often happens, the nurse makes it her business to turn the patient's room into a ventilating shaft for the foul air of the whole house. _Sick room airing the whole house._

An uninhabited room, a newly painted room,* an uncleaned closet or cupboard, may often become a reservoir of foul air for the whole house, because the person in charge never thinks of arranging that these places shall be always aired, always cleaned; she merely opens the window herself "when she goes in." _Uninhabited room fouling the whole house._

An agitating letter or message may be delivered, or an important letter or message _not_ delivered; a visitor whom it was of consequence to see, may be refused, or one whom it was of still more consequence _not_ to see may be admitted—because the person in charge has never asked herself this question, What is done when I am not there? † _Delivery and non-delivery of letters and messages._

At all events, one may safely say, a nurse cannot be with the

* That excellent paper, the _Builder_, mentions the lingering of the smell of paint for a month about a house as a proof of want of ventilation. Certainly— and, where there are ample windows to open, and these are never opened to get rid of the smell of paint, it is a proof of want of management in using the means of ventilation. Of course the smell will then remain for months. Why should it go? _Lingering smell of paint a want of care._

† Why should you let your patient ever be surprised, except by thieves? I do not know. In England, people do not come down the chimney, or through the window, unless they are thieves. They come in by the door, and somebody must open the door to them. The "somebody" charged with opening the door is one of two, three, or at most four persons. Why cannot these, at most, four persons be put in charge as to what is to be done when there is a ring at the door bell? _Why let your patient ever be surprised?_

The sentry at a post is changed much oftener than any servant at a private house or institution can possibly be. But what should we think of such an excuse as this: that the enemy had entered such a post because A and not B had been on guard? Yet I have constantly heard such an excuse made in the private house or institution and accepted: viz., that such a person had been "let in" or _not_ "let in," and such a parcel had been wrongly delivered or lost because A and not B had opened the door!

patient, open the door, eat her meals, take a message, all at one and the same time. Nevertheless the person in charge never seems to look the impossibility in the face.

Add to this that the *attempting* this impossibility does more to increase the poor Patient's hurry and nervousness than anything else.

Partial measures such as "being always in the way" yourself, increase instead of saving the patient's anxiety. Because they must be only partial. It is never thought that the patient remembers these things if you do not. He has not only to think whether the visit or letter may arrive, but whether you will be in the way at the particular day and hour when it may arrive. So that your *partial* measures for "being in the way" yourself, only increase the necessity for his thought. Whereas, if you could but arrange that the thing should always be done whether you are there or not, he need never think at all about it.

For the above reasons, whatever a patient *can* do for himself, it is better, *i.e.* less anxiety, for him to do for himself, unless the person in charge has the spirit of management.

It is evidently much less exertion for a patient to answer a letter for himself by return of post, than to have four conversations, wait five days, have six anxieties before it is off his mind, before the person who is to answer it has done so.

Apprehension, uncertainty, waiting, expectation, fear of surprise, do a patient more harm than any exertion. Remember, he is face to face with his enemy all the time, internally wrestling with him, having long imaginary conversations with him. You are thinking of something else. "Rid him of his adversary quickly," is a first rule with the sick.*

For the same reasons, always tell a patient and tell him beforehand when you are going out and when you will be back, whether it is for a day, an hour, or ten minutes. You fancy perhaps that it is better for him if he does not find out your going at all, better for him if you do not make yourself "of too much importance" to him; or else you cannot bear to give him the pain or the anxiety of the temporary separation.

No such thing. You *ought* to go, we will suppose. Health or duty requires it. Then say so to the patient openly. If you go without his knowing it, and he finds it out, he never will feel secure again that the things which depend upon you will be done when you are away, and in nine cases out of ten he will be right. If you go out without telling him when you will be back, he can take no measures nor precautions as to the things which concern you both, or which you do for him.

What is the cause of half the accidents which happen? If you look into the reports of trials or accidents, and especially of suicides, or into the medical history of fatal cases, it is almost incredible how often the whole thing turns upon something which

---

* There are many physical operations where *cæteris paribus* the danger is in a direct ratio to the time the operation lasts; and *cæteris paribus* the operator's success will be in direct ratio to his quickness. Now there are many mental operations where exactly the same rule holds good with the sick; *cæteris paribus* their capability of bearing such operations depends directly on the quickness, *without hurry*, with which they can be got through.

has happened because "he," or still oftener "she," "was not there." But it is still more incredible how often, how almost always this is accepted as a sufficient reason, a justification; why, the very fact of the thing having happened is the proof of its not being a justification. The person in charge was quite right not to be "*there*," he was called away for quite sufficient reason, or he was away for a daily recurring and unavoidable cause : yet no provision was made to supply his absence. The fault was not in his "being away," but in there being no management to supplement his "being away." When the sun is under a total eclipse or during his nightly absence, we light candles. But it would seem as if it did not occur to us that we must also supplement the person in charge of sick or of children, whether under an occasional eclipse or during a regular absence.

In institutions where many lives would be lost and the effect of such want of management would be terrible and patent, there is less of it than in the private house.*

Petty management better understood in institutions than in private houses.

* So true is this that I could mention two cases of women of very high position, both of whom died in the same way of the consequences of a surgical operation. And in both cases, I was told by the highest authority that the fatal result would not have happened in a London hospital.

But, as far as regards the art of petty management in hospitals, all the military hospitals I know must be excluded. Upon my own experience I stand, and I solemnly declare that I have seen or known of fatal accidents, such as suicides in *delirium tremens*, bleedings to death, dying patients dragged out of bed by drunken Medical Staff Corps men, and many other things less patent and striking, which would not have happened in London civil hospitals nursed by women. The medical officers should be absolved from all blame in these accidents. How can a medical officer mount guard all day and all night over a patient (say) in *delirium tremens ?* The fault lies in there being no organized system of attendance. Were a trustworthy *man* in charge of each ward, or set of wards, not as office clerk, but as head nurse, (and head nurse the best hospital serjeant, or ward master, is not now and cannot be, from default of the proper regulations), the thing would not, in all probability, have happened. But were a trustworthy *woman* in charge of the ward, or set of wards, the thing would not, in all certainty, have happened. In other words, it does not happen where a trustworthy woman is really in charge. And, in these remarks, I by no means refer only to exceptional times of great emergency in war hospitals, but also, and quite as much, to the ordinary run of military hospitals at home, in time of peace ; or to a time in war when our army was actually more healthy than at home in peace, and the pressure on our hospitals consequently much less.

What institutions are the exception?

It is often said that, in regimental hospitals, patients ought to "nurse each other," because the number of sick altogether being, say, but thirty, and out of these one only perhaps being seriously ill, and the other twenty-nine having little the matter with them, and nothing to do, they should be set to nurse the one ; also, that soldiers are so trained to obey, that they will be the most obedient, and therefore the best of nurses, add to which they are always kind to their comrades.

Nursing in Regimental Hospitals.

Now, have those who say this, considered that, in order to obey, you must know *how* to obey, and that these soldiers certainly do not know how to obey in nursing. I have seen these "kind" fellows (and how kind they are no one knows so well as myself) move a comrade so that, in one case at least, the man died in the act. I have seen the comrades' "kindness" produce abundance of spirits, to be drunk in secret. Let no one understand by this that female nurses ought to, or could be introduced in regimental hospitals. It would be most undesirable, even were it not impossible. But the **head** nurseship of a hospital

But in both, let whoever is in charge keep this simple question in her head (*not*, how can I always do this right thing myself, but) how can I provide for this right thing to be always done?

Then, when anything wrong has actually happened in consequence of her absence, which absence we will suppose to have been quite right, let her question still be (*not*, how can I provide against any more of such absences? which is neither possible nor desirable, but) how can I provide against any thing wrong arising out of my absence?

What it is to be "in charge." How few men, or even women, understand, either in great or in little things, what it is the being "in charge"—I mean, know how to carry out a "charge." From the most colossal calamities, down to the most trifling accidents, results are often traced (or rather *not* traced) to such want of some one "in charge" or of his knowing how to be "in charge." A short time ago the bursting of a funnel-casing on board the finest and strongest ship that ever was built, on her trial trip, destroyed several lives and put several hundreds in jeopardy—not from any undetected flaw in her new and untried works—but from a tap being closed which ought not to have been closed—from what every child knows would make its mother's tea-kettle burst. And this simply because no one seemed to know what it is to be "in charge," or *who* was in charge. Nay more, the jury at the inquest actually altogether ignored the same, and apparently considered the tap "in charge," for they gave as a verdict "accidental death."

This is the meaning of the word, on a large scale. On a much smaller scale, it happened, a short time ago, that an insane person burnt herself slowly and intentionally to death, while in her doctor's charge and almost in her nurse's presence. Yet neither was considered "at all to blame." The very fact of the accident happening proves its own case. There is nothing more to be said. Either they did not know their business or they did not know how to perform it.

To be "in charge" is certainly not only to carry out the proper measures yourself but to see that every one else does so too; to see that no one either wilfully or ignorantly thwarts or prevents such measures. It is neither to do everything yourself nor to appoint a number of people to each duty, but to ensure that each does that duty to which he is appointed. This is the meaning which must be attached to the word by (above all) those "in charge" of sick, whether of numbers or of individuals, (and indeed I think it is with individual sick that it is least understood. One sick person is often waited on by four with less precision, and is really less cared for than ten who are waited on by one; or at least than 40 who are waited on by 4; and all for want of this one person "in charge.)"

serjeant is the more essential, the more important, the more inexperienced the nurses. Undoubtedly, a London hospital "sister" does sometimes set relays of patients to watch a critical case; but, undoubtedly also, always under her own superintendence; and she is called to whenever there is something to be done, and she knows how to do it. The patients are not left to do it of their own unassisted genius, however "kind" and willing they may be.

It is often said that there are few good servants now : I say there are few good mistresses now. As the jury seems to have thought the tap was in charge of the ship's safety, so mistresses now seem to think the house is in charge of itself. They neither know how to give orders, nor how to teach their servants to obey orders—*i. e.* to obey intelligently, which is the real meaning of all discipline.

Again, people who are in charge often seem to have a pride in feeling that they will be "missed," that no one can understand or carry on their arrangements, their system, books, accounts, &c., but themselves. It seems to me that the pride is rather in carrying on a system, in keeping stores, closets, books, accounts, &c., so that any body can understand and carry them on—so that, in case of absence or illness, one can deliver every thing up to others and know that all will go on as usual, and that one shall never be missed.

NOTE.—It is often complained, that professional nurses, brought into private **Why hired** families, in case of sickness, make themselves intolerable by "ordering about" the **nurses give so** other servants, under plea of not neglecting the patient. Both things are true ; the **much trouble.** patient is often neglected, and the servants are often unfairly "put upon." But the fault is generally in the want of management of the head in charge. It is surely for her to arrange both that the nurse's place is, when necessary, supplemented, and that the patient is never neglected—things with a little management quite compatible, and indeed only attainable together. It is certainly not for the nurse to "order about" the servants.

IV. NOISE.

Unnecessary noise, or noise that creates an expectation in the **Unnecessary** mind, is that which hurts a patient. It is rarely the loudness of the **noise.** noise, the effect upon the organ of the ear itself, which appears to affect the sick. How well a patient will generally bear, *e. g.*, the putting up of a scaffolding close to the house, when he cannot bear the talking, still less the whispering, especially if it be of a familiar voice, outside his door.

There are certain patients, no doubt, especially where there is slight concussion or other disturbance of the brain, who are affected by mere noise. But intermittent noise, or sudden and sharp noise, in these as in all other cases, affects far more than continuous noise—noise with jar far more than noise without. Of one thing you may be certain, that anything which wakes a patient suddenly out of his sleep will invariably put him into a state of greater excitement, do him more serious, aye, and lasting mischief, than any continuous noise, however loud.

Never to allow a patient to be waked, intentionally or accident- **Never let a** ally, is a *sine quâ non* of all good nursing. If he is roused out of his **patient be** first sleep, he is almost certain to have no more sleep. It is a curious **waked out of** but quite intelligible fact that, if a patient is waked after a few **his first sleep.** hours' instead of a few minutes' sleep, he is much more likely to sleep again. Because pain, like irritability of brain, perpetuates and intensifies itself. If you have gained a respite of either in sleep you have gained more than the mere respite. Both the probability of recurrence and of the same intensity will be diminished; whereas both will be terribly increased by want of sleep. This is the reason why sleep is so all-important. This is the reason why a patient waked in the early part of his sleep loses not only his sleep, but his power to sleep. A healthy person who allows himself to sleep during the day will lose his sleep at night. But it is exactly the reverse with the sick generally; the more they sleep, the better will they be able to sleep.

Noise which excites expectation.

I have often been surprised at the thoughtlessness, (resulting in cruelty, quite unintentionally) of friends or of doctors who will hold a long conversation just in the room or passage adjoining to the room of the patient, who is either every moment expecting them to come in, or who has just seen them, and knows they are talking about him. If he is an amiable patient, he will try to occupy his attention elsewhere and not to listen—and this makes matters worse—for the strain upon his attention and the effort he makes are so great that it is well if he is not worse for hours

Whispered conversation in the room

after. If it is a whispered conversation in the same room, then it is absolutely cruel; for it is impossible that the patient's attention should not be involuntarily strained to hear. Walking on tip-toe, doing any thing in the room very slowly, are injurious, for exactly the same reasons. A firm light quick step, a steady quick hand are the desiderata; not the slow, lingering, shuffling foot, the timid, uncertain touch. Slowness is not gentleness, though it is often mistaken for such; quickness, lightness, and gentleness are quite compatible. Again, if friends and doctors did but watch, as nurses can and should watch, the features sharpening, the eyes growing almost wild, of fever patients who are listening for the entrance from the corridor of the persons whose voices they are hearing there, these would never run the risk again of creating such expectation, or irritation of mind.—Such unnecessary noise has undoubtedly induced or aggravated delirium in many cases. I have known such—in one case death ensued. It is but fair to say that this death was attributed to fright. It was the result of a long whispered conversation, within sight of the patient, about an impending operation; but any one who has known the more than stoicism, the cheerful coolness, with which the certainty of an operation will be accepted by any patient, capable of bearing an operation at all, if it is properly communicated to him, will hesitate to believe that it was mere fear which produced, as was averred, the fatal result in this instance. It was rather the uncertainty, the strained expectation as to what was to be decided upon.

Or just outside the door.

I need hardly say that the other common cause, namely, for a doctor or friend to leave the patient and communicate his opinion on the result of his visit to the friends just outside the patient's door, or in the adjoining room, after the visit, but within hearing or knowledge of the patient is, if possible, worst of all.

Noise of female dress.

It is, I think, alarming, peculiarly at this time, when the female ink-bottles are perpetually impressing upon us "woman's" "particular worth and general missionariness," to see that the dress of women is daily more and more unfitting them for any "mission," or usefulness at all. It is equally unfitted for all poetic and all domestic purposes. A man is now a more handy and far less objectionable being in a sick-room than a woman. Compelled by her dress, every woman now either shuffles or waddles—only a man can cross the floor of a sick-room without shaking it! What is become of woman's light step?—the firm, light, quick step we have been asking for?

Unnecessary noise, then, is the most cruel absence of care which can be inflicted either on sick or well. For, in all these remarks, the sick are only mentioned as suffering in a greater proportion than the well from precisely the same causes.

Unnecessary (although slight) noise injures a sick person much more than necessary noise (of a much greater amount).

All doctrines about mysterious affinities and aversions will be found to resolve themselves very much, if not entirely, into presence or absence of care in these things. *Patient's repulsion to nurses who rustle.*

A nurse who rustles (I am speaking of nurses professional and unprofessional) is the horror of a patient, though perhaps he does not know why.

The fidget of silk and of crinoline, the rattling of keys, the creaking of stays and of shoes, will do a patient more harm than all the medicines in the world will do him good.

The noiseless step of woman, the noiseless drapery of woman, are mere figures of speech in this day. Her skirts (and well if they do not throw down some piece of furniture) will at least brush against every article in the room as she moves.*

Again, one nurse cannot open the door without making everything rattle. Or she opens the door unnecessarily often, for want of remembering all the articles that might be brought in at once.

A good nurse will always make sure that no door or window in her patient's room shall rattle or creak; that no blind or curtain shall, by any change of wind through the open window, be made to flap—especially will she be careful of all this before she leaves her patients for the night. If you wait till your patients tell you, or remind you of these things, where is the use of their having a nurse? There are more shy than exacting patients, in all classes; and many

---

* Fortunate it is if her skirts do not catch fire—and if the nurse does not give herself up a sacrifice together with her patient, to be burnt in her own petticoats. *Burning of the crinolines.* I wish the Registrar-General would tell us the exact number of deaths by burning occasioned by this absurd and hideous custom. But if people will be stupid, let them take measures to protect themselves from their own stupidity—measures which every chemist knows, such as putting alum into starch, which prevents starched articles of dress from blazing up.

I wish too that people who wear crinoline could see the indecency of their own dress as other people see it. A respectable elderly woman stooping forward, invested in crinoline, exposes quite as much of her own person to the patient lying in the room as any opera dancer does on the stage. But no one will ever tell her this unpleasant truth. *Indecency of the crinolines.*

a patient passes a bad night, time after time, rather than remind his nurse every night of all the things she has forgotten.

If there are blinds to your windows, always take care to have them well up, when they are not being used. A little piece slipping down, and flapping with every draught, will distract a patient.

Hurry peculiarly hurtful to sick.
All hurry or bustle is peculiarly painful to the sick. And when a patient has compulsory occupations to engage him, instead of having simply to amuse himself, it becomes doubly injurious. The friend who remains standing and fidgetting about while a patient is talking business to him, or the friend who sits and proses, the one from an idea of not letting the patient talk, the other from an idea of amusing him,—each is equally inconsiderate. Always sit down when a sick person is talking business to you, show no signs of hurry, give complete attention and full consideration if your advice is wanted, and go away the moment the subject is ended.

How to visit the sick and not hurt them.
Always sit within the patient's view, so that when you speak to him he has not painfully to turn his head round in order to look at you. Everybody involuntarily looks at the person speaking. If you make this act a wearisome one on the part of the patient you are doing him harm. So also if by continuing to stand you make him continuously raise his eyes to see you. Be as motionless as possible, and never gesticulate in speaking to the sick.

Never make a patient repeat a message or request, especially if it be some time after. Occupied patients are often accused of doing too much of their own business. They are instinctively right. How often you hear the person, charged with the request of giving the message or writing the letter, say half an hour afterwards to the patient, " Did you appoint 12 o'clock ?" or, "What did you say was the address ?" or ask perhaps some much more agitating question— thus causing the patient the effort of memory, or worse still, of decision, all over again. It is really less exertion to him to write his letters himself. This is the almost universal experience of occupied invalids.

This brings us to another caution. Never speak to an invalid from behind, nor from the door, nor from any distance from him, nor when he is doing anything.

The official politeness of servants in these things is so grateful to invalids, that many prefer, without knowing why, having none but servants about them.

These things not fancy.
These things are not fancy. If we consider that, with sick as with well, every thought decomposes some nervous matter,—that decomposition as well as re-composition of nervous matter is always going on, and more quickly with the sick than with the well,—that, to obtrude abruptly another thought upon the brain while it is in the act of destroying nervous matter by thinking, is calling upon it to make a new exertion,—if we consider these things, which are facts, not fancies, we shall remember that we are doing positive injury by interrupting, by "startling a fanciful" person, as it is called. Alas! it is no fancy.

Interruption damaging to sick
If the invalid is forced, by his avocations, to continue occupations

requiring much thinking, the injury is doubly great. In feeding a patient suffering under delirium or stupor you may suffocate him, by giving him his food suddenly, but if you rub his lips gently with a spoon and thus attract his attention, he will swallow the food unconsciously, but with perfect safety. Thus it is with the brain. If you offer it a thought, especially one requiring a decision, abruptly, you do it a real not fanciful injury. Never speak to a sick person suddenly ; but, at the same time, do not keep his expectation on the tiptoe.

This rule, indeed, applies to the well quite as much as to the sick. And to well. I have never known persons who exposed themselves for years to constant interruption who did not muddle away their intellects by it at last. The process with them may be accomplished without pain. With the sick, pain gives warning of the injury.

Do not meet or overtake a patient who is moving about in order Keeping a patient standing. to speak to him, or to give him any message or letter. You might just as well give him a box on the ear. I have seen a patient fall flat on the ground who was standing when his nurse came into the room. This was an accident which might have happened to the most careful nurse. But the other is done with intention. A patient in such a state is not going to the East Indies. If you would wait ten seconds, or walk ten yards further, any promenade he could make would be over. You do not know the effort it is to a patient to remain standing for even a quarter of a minute to listen to you. If I had not seen the thing done by the kindest nurses and friends, I should have thought this caution quite superfluous.*

Patients are often accused of being able to " do much more when Patients dread surprise. nobody is by." It is quite true that they can. Unless nurses can be brought to attend to considerations of the kind of which we have given here but a few specimens, a very weak patient finds it really much less exertion to do things for himself than to ask for them. And he will, in order to do them, (very innocently and from instinct) calculate the time his nurse is likely to be absent, from a fear of her " coming in upon" him or speaking to him, just at the moment when he finds it quite as much as he can do to crawl from his bed to his chair, or from one room to another, or down stairs, or out of doors for a few minutes. Some extra call made upon his attention at that moment will quite upset him. In these cases you may be sure that a patient in the state we have described does not make such exertions more than once or twice a-day, and probably

---

* It is absolutely essential that a nurse should lay this down as a positive rule Never speak to a patient in the act of moving. to herself, never to speak to any patient who is standing or moving, as long as she exercises so little observation as not to know when a patient cannot bear it. I am satisfied that many of the accidents which happen from feeble patients tumbling down stairs, fainting after getting up, &c., happen solely from the nurse popping out of a door to speak to the patient just at that moment ; or from his fearing that she will do so. And that if the patient were even left to himself, till he can sit down, such accidents would much seldomer occur. If the nurse accompanies the patient let her not call upon him to speak. It is incredible that nurses cannot picture to themselves the strain upon the heart, the lungs, and the brain which the act of moving is to any feeble patient.

much about the same hour every day. And it is hard, indeed, if nurse and friends cannot calculate so as to let him make them undisturbed. Remember, that many patients can walk who cannot stand or even sit up. Standing is, of all positions, the most trying to a weak patient.

. Everything you do in a patient's room, after he is "put up" for the night, increases tenfold the risk of his having a bad night. But, if you rouse him up after he has fallen asleep, you do not risk, you secure him a bad night.

One hint I would give to all who attend or visit the sick, to all who have to pronounce an opinion upon sickness or its progress. Come back and look at your patient *after* he has had an hour's animated conversation with you. It is the best test of his real state we know. But never pronounce upon him from merely seeing what he does, or how he looks, during such a conversation. Learn also carefully and exactly, if you can, how he passed the night after it.

Effects of over-exertion on sick.

People rarely, if ever, faint while making an exertion. It is after it is over. Indeed, almost every effect of over-exertion appears after, not during such exertion. It is the highest folly to judge of the sick, as is so often done, when you see them merely during a period of excitement. People have very often died of that which, it has been proclaimed at the time, has " done them no harm."*

Remember never to lean against, sit upon, or unnecessarily shake, or even touch the bed in which a patient lies. This is invariably a painful annoyance. If you shake the chair on which he sits, he has a point by which to steady himself, in his feet. But on a bed or sofa, he is entirely at your mercy, and he feels every jar you give him all through him.

Difference between real and fancy patients.

In all that we have said, both here and elsewhere, let it be distinctly understood that we are not speaking of hypochondriacs. To distinguish between real and fancied disease forms an important branch of the education of a nurse. To manage fancy patients forms an important branch of her duties. But the nursing which real and that which fancied patients require is of different, or rather of opposite, character. And the latter will not be spoken of here. Indeed, many of the symptoms which are here mentioned are those which distinguish real from fancied disease.

Careless observation of the results of careless visits.

* As an old experienced nurse, I do most earnestly deprecate all such careless words. I have known patients delirious all night, after seeing a visitor who called them "better," thought they "only wanted a little amusement," and who came again, saying, "I hope you were not the worse for my visit," neither waiting for an answer, nor even looking at the case. No real patient will ever say, "Yes, but I was a great deal the worse."

It is not, however, either death or delirium of which, in these cases, there is most danger to the patient. Unperceived consequences are far more likely to ensue. *You* will have impunity—the poor patient will *not*. That is, the patient will suffer, although neither he nor the inflictor of the injury will attribute it to its real cause. It will not be directly traceable, except by a very careful observant nurse. The patient will often not even mention what has done him most harm.

It is true that hypochondriacs very often do that behind a nurse's back which they would not do before her face. Many such I have had as patients who scarcely ate anything at their regular meals; but if you concealed food for them in a drawer, they would take it at night or in secret. But this is from quite a different motive. They do it from the wish to conceal. Whereas the real patient will often boast to his nurse or doctor, if these do not shake their heads at him, of how much he has done, or eaten, or walked. To return to real disease.

Conciseness and decision are, above all things, necessary with the sick. Let your thought expressed to them be concisely and decidedly expressed. What doubt and hesitation there may be in your own mind must never be communicated to theirs, not even (I would rather say especially not) in little things. Let your doubt be to yourself, your decision to them. People who think outside their heads, the whole process of whose thought appears, like Homer's, in the act of secretion, who tell everything that led them towards this conclusion and away from that, ought never to be with the sick. *Conciseness necessary with Sick.*

Irresolution is what all patients most dread. Rather than meet this in others, they will collect all their data, and make up their minds for themselves. A change of mind in others, whether it is regarding an operation, or re-writing a letter, always injures the patient more than the being called upon to make up his mind to the most dreaded or difficult decision. Farther than this, in very many cases, the imagination in disease is far more active and vivid than it is in health. If you propose to the patient change of air to one place one hour, and to another the next, he has, in each case, immediately constituted himself in imagination the tenant of the place, gone over the whole premises in idea, and you have tired him as much by displacing his imagination, as if you had actually carried him over both places. *Irresolution most painful to them.*

Above all leave the sick room quickly and come into it quickly, not suddenly, not with a rush. But don't let the patient be wearily waiting for when you will be out of the room or when you will be in it. Conciseness and decision in your movements, as well as your words, are necessary in the sick room, as necessary as absence of hurry and bustle. To possess yourself entirely will ensure you from either failing—either loitering or hurrying.

If a patient has to see, not only to his own but also to his nurse's punctuality, or perseverance, or readiness, or calmness, to any or all of these things, he is far better without that nurse than with her— however valuable and handy her services may otherwise be to him, and however incapable he may be of rendering them to himself. *What a patient must not have to see to.*

With regard to reading aloud in the sick room, my experience is, that when the sick are too ill to read to themselves, they can seldom bear to be read to. Children, eye-patients, and uneducated persons are exceptions, or where there is any mechanical difficulty in reading. People who like to be read to, have generally not much the matter with them; while in fevers, or where there is much irritability of brain, the effort of listening to reading aloud has often *Reading aloud.*

brought on delirium. I speak with great diffidence; because there is an almost universal impression that it is *sparing* the sick to read aloud to them. But two things are certain :—

(1.) If there is some matter which *must* be read to a sick person, do it slowly. People often think that the way to get it over with least fatigue to him is to get it over in least time. They gabble; they plunge and gallop through the reading. There never was a greater mistake. Houdin, the conjuror, says that the way to make a story seem short is to tell it slowly. So it is with reading to the sick. I have often heard a patient say to such a mistaken reader, "Don't read it to me; tell it me."* Unconsciously he is aware that this will regulate the plunging, the reading with unequal paces, slurring over one part, instead of leaving it out altogether, if it is unimportant, and mumbling another. If the reader lets his own attention wander, and then stops to read up to himself, or finds he has read the wrong bit, then it is all over with the poor patient's chance of not suffering. Very few people know how to read to the sick; very few read aloud as pleasantly even as they speak. In reading they sing, they hesitate, they stammer, they hurry, they mumble; when in speaking they do none of these things. Reading aloud to the sick ought always to be rather slow, and exceedingly distinct, but not mouthing—rather monotonous, but not sing song —rather loud, but not noisy—and, above all, not too long. Be very sure of what your patient can bear.

(2.) The extraordinary habit of reading to oneself in a sick room, and reading aloud to the patient any bits which will amuse him or more often the reader, is unaccountably thoughtless. What *do* you think the patient is thinking of during your gaps of non-reading? Do you think that he amuses himself upon what you have read for precisely the time it pleases you to go on reading to yourself, and that his attention is ready for something else at precisely the time it pleases you to begin reading again? Whether the person thus read to be sick or well, whether he be doing nothing or doing something else while being thus read to, the self-absorption and want of observation of the person who does it, is equally difficult to understand— although very often the read*ee* is too amiable to say how much it disturbs him.

One thing more :—From the flimsy manner in which most modern houses are built, where every step on the stairs, and along the floors, is felt all over the house; the higher the story, the greater the vibration. It is inconceivable how much the sick suffer by having anybody overhead. In the solidly built old houses, which, fortunately, most hospitals are, the noise and shaking is comparatively trifling. But it is a serious cause of suffering, in lightly built houses, and with the irritability peculiar to some diseases. Better far put such patients at the top of the house, even with the additional fatigue of stairs, if you cannot secure the room above them being

* Sick children, if not too shy to speak, will always express this wish. They invariably prefer a story to be *told* to them, rather than read to them.

untenanted; you may otherwise bring on a state of restlessness which no opium will subdue. Do not neglect the warning, when a patient tells you that he " Feels every step above him to cross his heart." Remember that every noise a patient cannot *see* partakes of the character of suddenness to him; and I am persuaded that patients with these peculiarly irritable nerves, are positively less injured by having persons in the same room with them than overhead, or separated by only a thin compartment. Any sacrifice to secure silence for these cases is worth while, because no air, however good, no attendance, however careful, will do anything for such cases without quiet.

NOTE.—The effect of music upon the sick has been scarcely at all noticed. Music. In fact, its expensiveness, as it is now, makes any general application of it quite out of the question. I will only remark here, that wind instruments, including the human voice, and stringed instruments, capable of continuous sound, have generally a beneficent effect—while the piano-forte, with such instruments as have *no* continuity of sound, has just the reverse. The finest piano-forte playing will damage the sick, while an air, like " Home, sweet home," or " Assisa a piè d'un salice," on the most ordinary grinding organ will sensibly soothe them—and this quite independent of association.

V. VARIETY.

To any but an old nurse, or an old patient, the degree would be quite inconceivable to which the nerves of the sick suffer from seeing the same walls, the same ceiling, the same surroundings during a long confinement to one or two rooms. Variety a means of recovery.

The superior cheerfulness of persons suffering severe paroxysms of pain over that of persons suffering from nervous debility has often been remarked upon, and attributed to the enjoyment of the former of their intervals of respite. I incline to think that the majority of cheerful cases is to be found among those patients who are not confined to one room, whatever their suffering, and that the majority of depressed cases will be seen among those subjected to a long monotony of objects about them.

The nervous frame really suffers as much from this as the digestive organs from long monotony of diet, as *e.g.* the soldier from his twenty-one years' " boiled beef."

The effect in sickness of beautiful objects, of variety of objects, and especially of brilliancy of colour is hardly at all appreciated. Colour and form means of recovery.

Such cravings are usually called the " fancies " of patients. And often doubtless patients have "fancies," as, *e.g.* when they desire two contradictions. But much more often, their (so called)"fancies" are the most valuable indications of what is necessary for their recovery. And it would be well if nurses would watch these (so called) "fancies" closely.

I have seen, in fevers (and felt, when I was a fever patient myself) the most acute suffering produced from the patient (in a hut) not being able to see out of window, and the knots in the wood

D

being the only view. I shall never forget the rapture of fever patients over a bunch of bright-coloured flowers. I remember (in my own case) a nosegay of wild flowers being sent me, and from that moment recovery becoming more rapid.

This is no fancy. People say the effect is only on the mind. It is no such thing. The effect is on the body, too. Little as we know about the way in which we are affected by form, by colour, and light, we do know this, that they have an actual physical effect.

Variety of form and brilliancy of colour in the objects presented to patients are actual means of recovery.

But it must be *slow* variety, e.g., if you shew a patient ten or twelve engravings successively, ten-to-one that he does not become cold and faint, or feverish, or even sick; but hang one up opposite him, one on each successive day, or week, or month, and he will revel in the variety.

Flowers. The folly and ignorance which reign too often supreme over the sick-room, cannot be better exemplified than by this. While the nurse will leave the patient stewing in a corrupting atmosphere, the best ingredient of which is carbonic acid; she will deny him, on the plea of unhealthiness, a glass of cut-flowers, or a growing plant. Now, no one ever saw "overcrowding" by plants in a room or ward. And the carbonic acid they give off at nights would not poison a fly. Nay, in overcrowded rooms, they actually absorb carbonic acid and give off oxygen. Cut-flowers also decompose water and produce oxygen gas. It is true there are certain flowers, e.g., lilies, the smell of which is said to depress the nervous system. These are easily known by the smell, and can be avoided.

Effect of body on mind. Volumes are now written and spoken upon the effect of the mind upon the body. Much of it is true. But I wish a little more was thought of the effect of the body on the mind. You who believe yourselves overwhelmed with anxieties, but are able every day to walk up Regent-street, or out in the country, to take your meals with others in other rooms, &c., &c., you little know how much your anxieties are thereby lightened; you little know how intensified they become to those who can have no change;* how the very walls of their sick rooms seem hung with their cares; how the ghosts of their troubles haunt their beds; how impossible it is for them to escape from a pursuing thought without some help from variety.

A patient can just as much move his leg when it is fractured as change his thoughts when no external help from variety is given him. This is, indeed, one of the main sufferings of sickness; just

Sick suffer to excess from mental as well as bodily pain. * It is a matter of painful wonder to the sick themselves how much painful ideas predominate over pleasurable ones in their impressions; they reason with themselves; they think themselves ungrateful; it is all of no use. The fact is, that these painful impressions are far better dismissed by a real laugh, if you can excite one by books or conversation, than by any direct reasoning; or if the patient is too weak to laugh, some impression from nature is what he wants. I have mentioned the cruelty of letting him stare at a dead wall. In many diseases, especially in convalescence from fever, that wall will appear to make all sorts of faces at him; now flowers never do this. Form, colour, will free your patient from his painful ideas better than any argument.

as the fixed posture is one of the main sufferings of the broken limb.

It is an ever recurring wonder to see educated people, who call themselves nurses, acting thus. They vary their own objects, their own employments many times a day; and while nursing (!) some bed-ridden sufferer, they let him lie there staring at a dead wall, without any change of object to enable him to vary his thoughts; and it never even occurs to them, at least to move his bed so that he can look out of window. No, the bed is to be always left in the darkest, dullest, remotest, part of the room.* *Help the sick to vary their thoughts.*

I think it is a very common error among the well to think that "with a little more self-control" the sick might, if they choose, "dismiss painful thoughts" which "aggravate their disease," &c. Believe me, almost *any* sick person, who behaves decently well, exercises more self-control every moment of his day than you will ever know till you are sick yourself. Almost every step that crosses his room is painful to him; almost every thought that crosses his brain is painful to him; and if he can speak without being savage, and look without being unpleasant, he is exercising self-control.

Suppose you have been up all night, and instead of being allowed to have your cup of tea, you were to be told that you ought to "exercise self-control," what should you say? Now, the nerves of the sick are always in the state that yours are in after you have been up all night.

We will suppose the diet of the sick to be cared for. Then, this state of nerves is most frequently to be relieved by care in affording them a pleasant view, a judicious variety as to flowers,† and pretty things. Light by itself will often relieve it. The craving for "the return of day," which the sick so constantly evince, is generally nothing but the desire for light, the remembrance of the relief which a variety of objects before the eye affords to the harassed sick mind. *Supply to the sick the defect of manual labour.*

Again, every man and every woman has some amount of manual employment, excepting a few fine ladies, who do not even dress themselves, and who are virtually in the same category, as to nerves, as the sick. Now, you can have no idea of the relief which manual labour is to you—of the degree to which the deprivation of manual

---

* I remember a case in point. A man received an injury to the spine, from an accident, which after a long confinement ended in death. He was a workman —had not in his composition a single grain of what is called "enthusiasm for nature,"—but he was desperate to "see once more out of window." His nurse actually got him on her back, and managed to perch him up at the window for an instant, "to see out." The consequence to the poor nurse was a serious illness, which nearly proved fatal. The man never knew it; but a great many other people did. Yet the consequence in none of their minds, so far as I know, was the conviction that the craving for variety in the starving eye, is just as desperate as that for food in the starving stomach, and tempts the famishing creature in either case to steal for its satisfaction. No other word will express it but "desperation." And it sets the seal of ignorance and stupidity just as much on the governors and attendants of the sick if they do not provide the sick-bed with a "view" of some kind, as if they did not provide the hospital with a kitchen. *Desperate desire in the sick to "see out of window."*

† No one who has watched the sick can doubt the fact, that some feel stimulus from looking at scarlet flowers, exhaustion from looking at deep blue, &c. *Physical effect of colour.*

D 2

employment increases the peculiar irritability from which many sick suffer.

A little needle-work, a little writing, a little cleaning, would be the greatest relief the sick could have, if they could do it; these *are* the greatest relief to you, though you do not know it. Reading, though it is often the only thing the sick can do, is not this relief. Bearing this in mind, bearing in mind that you have all these varieties of employment which the sick cannot have, bear also in mind to obtain for them all the varieties which they can enjoy.

I need hardly say that I am well aware that excess in needle-work, in writing, in any other continuous employment, will produce the same irritability that defect in manual employment (as one cause) produces in the sick.

VI. TAKING FOOD.

Want of attention to hours of taking food.

Every careful observer of the sick will agree in this that thousands of patients are annually starved in the midst of plenty, from want of attention to the ways which alone make it possible for them to take food. This want of attention is as remarkable in those who urge upon the sick to do what is quite impossible to them, as in the sick themselves who will not make the effort to do what is perfectly possible to them.

For instance, to the large majority of very weak patients it is quite impossible to take any solid food before 11 A.M., nor then, if their strength is still further exhausted by fasting till that hour. For weak patients have generally feverish nights and, in the morning, dry mouths; and, if they could eat with those dry mouths, it would be the worse for them. A spoonful of beef-tea, of arrowroot and wine, of egg flip, every hour, will give them the requisite nourishment, and prevent them from being too much exhausted to take at a later hour the solid food, which is necessary for their recovery. And every patient who can swallow at all can swallow these liquid things, if he chooses. But how often do we hear a mutton-chop, an egg, a bit of bacon, ordered to a patient for breakfast, to whom (as a moment's consideration would show us) it must be quite impossible to masticate such things at that hour.

Again, a nurse is ordered to give a patient a tea-cup full of some article of food every three hours. The patient's stomach rejects it. If so, try a table-spoon full every hour; if this will not do, a tea-spoon full every quarter of an hour.

I am bound to say, that I think more patients are lost by want of care and ingenuity in these momentous minutiæ in private nursing than in public hospitals. And I think there is more of the *entente cordiale* to assist one another's hands between the doctor and his head nurse in the latter institutions, than between the doctor and the patient's friends in the private house.

Life often hangs upon minutes in taking food.

If we did but know the consequences which may ensue, in very weak patients, from ten minutes' fasting or repletion, (I call it repletion when they are obliged to let too small an interval elapse between taking food and some other exertion, owing to the nurse's unpunctuality), we should be more careful never to let this occur. In very weak patients there is often a nervous difficulty of swallowing, which is so much increased by any other call upon their strength that, unless they have their food punctually at the minute, which minute again must be arranged so as to fall in with no other minute's occupation, they can take nothing till the next respite occurs—so that an unpunctuality or delay of ten minutes may very well turn out to be one of two or three hours. And why is it not as easy to be punctual to a minute? Life often literally hangs upon these minutes.

In acute cases, where life or death is to be determined in a few hours, these matters are very generally attended to, especially in Hospitals ; and the number of cases is large where the patient is, as it were, brought back to life by exceeding care on the part of the Doctor or Nurse, or both, in ordering and giving nourishment with minute selection and punctuality.

But, in chronic cases, lasting over months and years, where the fatal issue is often determined at last by mere protracted starvation, I had rather not enumerate the instances which I have known where a little ingenuity, and a great deal of perseverance, might, in all probability, have averted the result. The consulting the hours when the patient can take food, the observation of the times, often varying, when he is most faint, the altering seasons of taking food, in order to anticipate and prevent such times—all this, which requires observation, ingenuity, and perseverance (and these really constitute the good Nurse), might save more lives than we wot of. *Patients often starved to death in chronic cases.*

To leave the patient's untasted food by his side, from meal to meal, in hopes that he will eat it in the interval, is simply to prevent him from taking any food at all. I have known patients literally incapacitated from taking one article of food after another, by this piece of ignorance. Let the food come at the right time, and be taken away, eaten or uneaten, at the right time; but never let a patient have " something always standing " by him, if you don't wish to disgust him of everything. *Food never to be left by the patient's side.*

On the other hand, I have known a patient's life saved (he was sinking for want of food) by the simple question, put to him by the doctor, " But is there no hour when you feel you could eat?" " Oh, yes," he said, " I could always take something at — o'clock and — o'clock." The thing was tried and succeeded. Patients very seldom, however, can tell this ; it is for you to watch and find it out.

A patient should, if possible, not see or smell either the food of others, or a greater amount of food than he himself can consume at one time, or even hear food talked about or see it in the raw state. I know of no exception to the above rule. The breaking of it always induces a greater or less incapacity of taking food. *Patient had better not see more food than his own.*

In hospital wards it is of course impossible to observe all this ; and in single wards, where a patient must be continuously and closely watched, it is frequently impossible to relieve the attendant, so that his or her own meals can be taken out of the ward. But it is not the less true that, in such cases, even where the patient is not himself aware of it, his possibility of taking food is limited by seeing the attendant eating meals under his observation. In some cases the sick are aware of it, and complain. A case where the patient was supposed to be insensible, but complained as soon as able to speak, is now present to my recollection.

Remember, however, that the extreme punctuality in well-ordered hospitals, the rule that nothing shall be done in the ward while the patients are having their meals, go far to counterbalance what unavoidable evil there is in having patients together. I have often seen the private nurse go on dusting or fidgeting about in a sick room all the while the patient is eating, or trying to eat.

That the more alone an invalid can be when taking food, the better, is unquestionable; and, even if he must be fed, the nurse should not allow him to talk, or talk to him, especially about food, while eating.

When a person is compelled, by the pressure of occupation, to continue his business while sick, it ought to be a rule WITHOUT ANY EXCEPTION WHATEVER, that no one shall bring business to him or talk to him while he is taking food, nor go on talking to him on interesting subjects up to the last moment before his meals, nor make an engagement with him immediately after, so that there be any hurry of mind while taking them.

Upon the observance of these rules, especially the first, often depends the patient's capability of taking food at all, or, if he is amiable and forces himself to take food, of deriving any nourishment from it.

You cannot be too careful as to quality in sick diet.
A nurse should never put before a patient milk that is sour, meat or soup that is turned, an egg that is bad, or vegetables underdone. Yet often I have seen these things brought in to the sick in a state perfectly perceptible to every nose or eye except the nurse's. It is here that the clever nurse appears ; she will not bring in the peccant article, but, not to disappoint the patient, she will whip up something else in a few minutes. Remember that sick cookery should half do the work of your poor patient's weak digestion. But if you further impair it with your bad articles, I know not what is to become of him or of it.

If the nurse is an intelligent being, and not a mere carrier of diets to and from the patient, let her exercise her intelligence in these things. How often we have known a patient eat nothing at all in the day, because one meal was left untasted (at that time he was incapable of eating), at another the milk was sour, the third was spoiled by some other accident. And it never occurred to the nurse to extemporize some expedient,—it never occurred to her that as he had had no solid food that day, he might eat a bit of toast (say) with his tea in the evening, or he might have some meal an hour earlier. A patient who cannot touch his dinner at two, will often accept it gladly, if brought to him at seven. But somehow nurses never "think of these things." One would imagine they did not consider themselves bound to exercise their judgment; they leave it to the patient. Now I am quite sure that it is better for a patient rather to suffer these neglects than to try to teach his nurse to nurse him, if she does not know how. It ruffles him, and if he is ill he is in no condition·to teach, especially upon himself. The above remarks apply much more to private nursing than to hospitals.

I would say to the nurse, have a rule of thought about your patient's diet; consider, remember how much he has had, and how much he ought to have to·day. Generally, the only rule of the private patient's diet is what the nurse has to give. It is true she cannot give him what she has not got; but his stomach does not wait for her convenience, or even her necessity.* If it is used to having its stimulus at one hour to-day, and to-morrow it does not have it, because she has failed in getting it, he will suffer. She must be always exercising her ingenuity to supply defects, and to remedy accidents which will happen among the best contrivers, but from which the patient does not suffer the less, because "they cannot be helped." *Nurse must have some rule of thought about her patient's diet.*

One very minute caution,—take care not to spill into your patient's saucer, in other words, take care that the outside bottom rim of his cup shall be quite dry and clean; if, every time he lifts his cup to his lips, he has to carry the saucer with it, or else to drop the liquid upon, and to soil his sheet, or his bed-gown, or pillow, or if he is sitting up, his dress, you have no idea what a difference this minute want of care on your part makes to his comfort and even to his willingness for food *Keep your patient's cup dry underneath.*

VII.   WHAT FOOD?

I will mention one or two of the most common errors among women in charge of sick respecting sick diet. One is the belief that beef tea is the most nutritive of all articles. Now, just try and boil down a lb. of beef into beef tea, evaporate your beef tea, and see what is left of your beef. You will find that there is barely a tea-spoonful of solid nourishment to half a pint of water in beef tea;—never-theless there is a certain reparative quality in it, we do not know what, as there is in tea;—but it may safely be given in almost any inflammatory disease, and is as little to be depended upon with the healthy or convalescent where much nourishment is required. Again, it is an ever ready saw that an egg is equivalent to a lb. of meat,—whereas it is not at all so. Also, it is seldom noticed with how many *Common errors in diet.* *Beef tea.*

* Why, because the nurse has not got some food to-day which the patient takes, can the patient wait four hours for food to-day, who could not wait two hours yester-day? Yet this is the only logic one generally hears. On the other hand, the other logic, viz., of the nurse giving a patient a thing because she *has* got it, is equally fatal. If she happens to have fresh jelly, or fresh fruit, she will frequently give it to the patient half-an-hour after his dinner, or at his dinner, when he cannot possibly eat that and the broth too—or worse still leave it by his bed-side till he is so sickened with the sight of it, that he cannot eat it at all. *Nurse must have some rule of time about the patient's diet.*

Eggs.

patients, particularly of nervous or bilious temperament, eggs disagree. All puddings made with eggs, are distasteful to them in consequence. An egg, whipped up with wine, is often the only form in which they can take this kind of nourishment. Again, if the patient has attained to eating meat, it is supposed that to give him meat is the only thing needful for his recovery; whereas scorbutic sores have been actually known to appear among sick persons living in the midst of plenty in England, which could be traced to no other source than this, viz.: that the nurse, depending on meat alone, had allowed the patient to be without vegetables for a considerable time, these latter being so badly cooked that he always left them untouched.

Meat without vegetables.

Arrowroot.

Arrowroot is another grand dependence of the nurse. As a vehicle for wine, and as a restorative quickly prepared, it is all very well. But it is nothing but starch and water. Flour is both more nutritive, and less liable to ferment, and is preferable wherever it can be used.

Milk, butter, cream, &c.

Again, milk and the preparations from milk, are a most important article of food for the sick. Butter is the lightest kind of animal fat, and though it wants the sugar and some of the other elements which there are in milk, yet it is most valuable both in itself and in enabling the patient to eat more bread. Flour, oats, groats, barley, and their kind, are as we have already said, preferable in all their preparations to all the preparations of arrow root, sago, tapioca, and their kind. Cream, in many long chronic diseases, is quite irreplaceable by any other article whatever. It seems to act in the same manner as beef tea, and to most it is much easier of digestion than milk. In fact, it seldom disagrees. Cheese is not usually digestible by the sick, but it is pure nourishment for repairing waste; and I have seen sick, and not a few either, whose craving for cheese shewed how much it was needed by them.*

But, if fresh milk is so valuable a food for the sick, the least change or sourness in it, makes it of all articles, perhaps, the most injurious; diarrhœa is a common result of fresh milk allowed to become at all sour. The nurse therefore ought to exercise her utmost care in this. In large institutions for the sick, even the poorest, the utmost care is exercised. Wenham Lake ice is used for this express purpose every summer, while the private patient, perhaps, never tastes a drop of milk that is not sour, all through the hot weather, so little does the private nurse understand the necessity of such care. Yet, if you consider that the only drop of real nourishment in your patient's tea is the drop of milk, and how much almost all English patients depend

Intelligent cravings of particular sick for particular articles of diet.

* In the diseases produced by bad food, such as scorbutic dysentery and diarrhœa, the patient's stomach often craves for and digests things, some of which certainly would be laid down in no dietary that ever was invented for sick, and especially not for such sick. These are fruit, pickles, jams, gingerbread, fat of ham or of bacon, suet, cheese, butter, milk. These cases I have seen not by ones, nor by tens, but by hundreds. And the patient's stomach was right and the book was wrong. The articles craved for, in these cases, might have been principally arranged under the two heads of fat and vegetable acids. There is often a marked difference between men and women in this matter of sick feeding. Women's digestion is generally slower.

upon their tea, you will see the great importance of not depriving your patient of this drop of milk. Buttermilk, a totally different thing, is often very useful, especially in fevers.

In laying down rules of diet, by the amounts of "solid nutri- *Sweet things.* ment" in different kinds of food, it is constantly lost sight of what the patient requires to repair his waste, what he can take and what he can't. You cannot diet a patient from a book, you cannot make up the human body as you would make up a prescription,—so many parts "carboniferous," so many parts "nitrogenous" will consti- tute a perfect diet for the patient. The nurse's observation here will materially assist the doctor—the patient's "fancies" will materially assist the nurse. For instance, sugar is one of the most nutritive of all articles, being pure carbon, and is particularly recom- mended in some books. But the vast majority of all patients in England, young and old, male and female, rich and poor, hospital and private, dislike sweet things,—and while I have never known a person take to sweets when he was ill who disliked them when he was well, I have known many fond of them when in health, who in sickness would leave off anything sweet, even to sugar in tea,—sweet puddings, sweet drinks, are their aversion; the furred tongue almost always likes what is sharp or pungent. Scorbutic patients are an exception, they often crave for sweetmeats and jams.

Jelly is another article of diet in great favour with nurses and *Jelly.* friends of the sick; even if it could be eaten solid, it would not nourish, but it is simply the height of folly to take ⅓ oz. of gelatine and make it into a certain bulk by dissolving it in water and then to give it to the sick, as if the mere bulk represented nourishment. It is now known that jelly does not nourish, that it has a tendency to produce diarrhœa,—and to trust to it to repair the waste of a diseased constitution is simply to starve the sick under the guise of feeding them. If 100 spoonfuls of jelly were given in the course of the day, you would have given one spoonful of gelatine, which spoonful has no nutritive power whatever.

And, nevertheless, gelatine contains a large quantity of nitrogen, which is one of the most powerful elements in nutrition; on the other hand, beef tea may be chosen as an illustration of great nutrient power in sickness, co-existing with a very small amount of solid nitrogenous matter.

Dr. Christison says that "every one will be struck with the readi- *Beef tea.* ness with which" certain classes of "patients will often take diluted meat juice or beef tea repeatedly, when they refuse all other kinds of food." This is particularly remarkable in "cases of gastric fever, in which," he says, "little or nothing else besides beef tea or diluted meat juice" has been taken for weeks or even months, "and yet a pint of beef tea contains scarcely ¼ oz. of anything but water,"—the result is so striking that he asks what is its mode of action? "Not simply nutrient—¼ oz. of the most nutritive material cannot nearly replace the daily wear and tear of the tissues in any circumstances. Possibly," he says, "it belongs to a new denomination of remedies."

It has been observed that a small quantity of beef tea added to other articles of nutrition augments their power out of all proportion to the additional amount of solid matter.

The reason why jelly should be innutritious and beef tea nutritious to the sick, is a secret yet undiscovered, but it clearly shows that careful observation of the sick is the only clue to the best dietary.

Observation, not chemistry, must decide sick diet. Chemistry has as yet afforded little insight into the dieting of sick. All that chemistry can tell us is the amount of " carboniferous " or " nitrogenous " elements. discoverable in different dietetic articles. It has given us lists of dietetic substances, arranged in the order of their richness in one or other of these principles; but that is all. In the great majority of cases, the stomach of the patient is guided by other principles of selection than merely the amount of carbon or nitrogen in the diet. No doubt, in this as in other things, nature has very definite rules for her guidance, but these rules can only be ascertained by the most careful observation at the bed-side. She there teaches us that living chemistry, the chemistry of reparation, is something different from the chemistry of the laboratory. Organic chemistry is useful, as all knowledge is, when we come face to face with nature; but it by no means follows that we should learn in the laboratory any one of the reparative processes going on in disease.

Again, the nutritive power of milk and of the preparations from milk, is very much undervalued; there is nearly as much nourishment in half a pint of milk as there is in a quarter of a lb. of meat. But this is not the whole question or nearly the whole. The main question is what the patient's stomach can assimilate or derive nourishment from, and of this the patient's stomach is the sole judge. Chemistry cannot tell this. The patient's stomach must be its own chemist. The diet which will keep the healthy man healthy, will kill the sick one. The same beef which is the most nutritive of all meat and which nourishes the healthy man, is the least nourishing of all food to the sick man, whose half-dead stomach can *assimilate* no part of it, that is, make no food out of it. On a diet of beef tea healthy men on the other hand speedily lose their strength.

Home-made bread. I have known patients live for many months without touching bread, because they could not eat baker's bread. These were mostly country patients, but not all. Home-made bread or brown bread is a most important article of diet for many patients. The use of aperients may be entirely superseded by it. Oat cake is another.

Sound observation has scarcely yet been brought to bear on sick diet. To watch for the opinions, then, which the patient's stomach gives, rather than to read " analyses of foods," is the business of all those who have to settle what the patient is to eat—perhaps the most important thing to be provided for him after the air he is to breathe. Now the medical man who sees the patient only once a day or even only once or twice a week, cannot possibly tell this without the assistance of the patient himself, or of those who are in constant observation on the patient. The utmost the medical man can tell is whether the patient is weaker or stronger at this visit than he was at the last visit. I should therefore say that incomparably the most important office of the nurse, after she has taken care of the patient's air, is to take care to observe the effect of his food, and report it to the medical attendant.

It is quite incalculable the good that would certainly come from such *sound* and close observation in this almost neglected branch of nursing, or the help it would give to the medical man.

A great deal too much against tea* is said by wise people, and a great deal too much of tea is given to the sick by foolish people. When you see the natural and almost universal craving in English sick for their " tea," you cannot but feel that nature knows what she is about. But a little tea or coffee restores them quite as much as a great deal, and a great deal of tea and especially of coffee impairs the little power of digestion they have. Yet a nurse because she sees how one or two cups of tea or coffee restores her patient, thinks that three or four cups will do twice as much. This is not the case at all; it is however certain that there is nothing yet discovered which is a substitute to the English patient for his cup of tea; he can take it when he can take nothing else, and he often can't take anything else if he has it not. I should be very glad if any of the abusers of tea would point out what to give to an English patient after a sleepless night, instead of tea. If you give it at 5 or 6 o'clock in the morning, he may even sometimes fall asleep after it, and get perhaps his only two or three hours' sleep during the twenty-four. At the same time you never should give tea or coffee to the sick, as a rule, after 5 o'clock in the afternoon. Sleeplessness in the early night is from excitement generally and is increased by tea or coffee; sleeplessness which continues to the early morning is from exhaustion often, and is relieved by tea. The only English patients I have ever known refuse tea, have been typhus cases, and the first sign of their getting better was their craving again for tea. In general, the dry and dirty tongue always prefers tea to coffee, and will quite decline milk, unless with tea. Coffee is a better restorative than tea, but a

Tea and coffee.

---

* It is made a frequent recommendation to persons about to incur great exhaustion, either from the nature of the service or from their being not in a state fit for it, to eat a piece of bread before they go. I wish the recommenders would themselves try the experiment of substituting a piece of bread for a cup of tea or coffee or beef tea as a refresher. They would find it a very poor comfort. When soldiers have to set out fasting on fatiguing duty, when nurses have to go fasting in to their patients, it is a hot restorative they want, and ought to have, before they go, not a cold bit of bread. And dreadful have been the consequences of neglecting this. If they can take a bit of bread *with* the hot cup of tea, so much the better, but not *instead* of it. The fact that there is more nourishment in bread than in almost anything else has probably induced the mistake. That it is a fatal mistake there is no doubt. It seems, though very little is known on the subject, that what "assimilates" itself directly and with the least trouble of digestion with the human body is the best for the above circumstances. Bread requires two or three processes of assimilation, before it becomes like the human body.

The almost universal testimony of English men and women who have undergone great fatigue, such as riding long journeys without stopping, or sitting up for several nights in succession, is that they could do it best upon an occasional cup of tea—and nothing else.

Let experience, not theory, decide upon this as upon all other things.

greater impairer of the digestion. Let the patient's taste decide. You will say that, in cases of great thirst, the patient's craving decides that it will drink *a great deal* of tea, and that you cannot help it. But in these cases be sure that the patient requires diluents for quite other purposes than quenching the thirst; he wants a great deal of some drink, not only of tea, and the doctor will order what he is to have, barley water or lemonade, or soda water and milk, as the case may be.

Lehmann, quoted by Dr. Christison, says that, among the well and active "the infusion of 1 oz. of roasted coffee daily will diminish the waste" going on in the body "by one-fourth," and Dr. Christison adds that tea has the same property. Now this is actual experiment. Lehmann weighs the man and finds the fact from his weight. It is not deduced from any "analysis" of food. All experience among the sick shows the same thing.*

Cocoa. Cocoa is often recommended to the sick in lieu of tea or coffee. But independently of the fact that English sick very generally dislike cocoa, it has quite a different effect from tea or coffee. It is an oily starchy nut having no restorative power at all, but simply increasing fat. It is pure mockery of the sick, therefore, to call it a substitute for tea. For any renovating stimulus it has, you might just as well offer them chesnuts instead of tea.

Bulk. An almost universal error among nurses is in the bulk of the food and especially the drinks they offer to their patients Suppose a patient ordered 4 oz. brandy during the day, how is he to take this if you make it into four pints with diluting it ? The same with tea and beef tea, with arrowroot, milk, &c. You have not increased the nourishment, you have not increased the renovating power of these articles, by increasing their bulk,—you have very likely diminished both by giving the patient's digestion more to do, and most likely of all, the patient will leave half of what he has been ordered to take, because he cannot swallow the bulk with which you have been pleased to invest it. It requires very nice observation and care (and meets with hardly any) to determine what will not be too thick or strong for the patient to take, while giving him no more than the bulk which he is able to swallow.

* In making coffee, it is absolutely necessary to buy it in the berry and grind it at home. Otherwise you may reckon upon its containing a certain amount of chicory, *at least.* This is not a question of the taste or of the wholesomeness of chicory. It is that chicory has nothing at all of the properties for which you give coffee. And therefore you may as well not give it.

Again, all laundresses, mistresses of dairy-farms, head nurses (I speak of the good old sort only—women who unite a good deal of hard manual labour with the head-work necessary for arranging the day's business, so that none of it shall tread upon the heels of something else) set great value, I have observed, upon having a high-priced tea. This is called extravagant. But these women are "extravagant" in nothing else. And they are right in this. Real tea-leaf tea alone contains the restorative they want; which is not to be found in sloe-leaf tea.

The mistresses of houses, who cannot even go over their own house once a-day, are incapable of judging for these women. For they are incapable themselves, to all appearance, of the spirit of arrangement (no small task) necessary for managing a large ward or dairy.

VIII. BED AND BEDDING.

A few words upon bedsteads and bedding; and principally as Feverishness regards patients who are entirely, or almost entirely, confined to bed. a symptom of
Feverishness is generally supposed to be a symptom of fever— bedding. in nine cases out of ten it is a symptom of bedding.* The patient has had re-introduced into the body the emanations from himself which day after day and week after week saturate his unaired bedding. How can it be otherwise? Look at the ordinary bed in which a patient lies.

If I were looking out for an example in order to show what *not* Uncleanliness to do, I should take the specimen of an ordinary bed in a private of ordinary house: a wooden bedstead, two or even three mattresses piled up to bedding. above the height of a table; a vallance attached to the frame— nothing but a miracle could ever thoroughly dry or air such a bed and bedding. The patient must inevitably alternate between cold damp after his bed is made, and warm damp before, both saturated with organic matter,† and this from the time the mattresses are put under him till the time they are picked to pieces, if this is ever done.

If you consider that an adult in health exhales by the lungs and Air your dirty skin in the twenty-four hours three pints at least of moisture, loaded sheets, not with organic matter ready to enter into putrefaction; that in sickness only your the quantity is often greatly increased, the quality is always more clean ones. noxious—just ask yourself next where does all this moisture go to? Chiefly into the bedding, because it cannot go anywhere else. And it stays there; because, except perhaps a weekly change of sheets, scarcely any other airing is attempted. A nurse will be careful to fidgetiness about airing the clean sheets from clean damp, but airing the dirty sheets from noxious damp will never even occur to her. Besides this, the most dangerous effluvia we know of are from the excreta of the sick—these are placed, at least temporarily, where they must throw their effluvia into the under side of the bed, and the space under the bed is never aired; it cannot be, with our arrangements. Must not such a bed be always saturated, and be always the means of re-introducing into the system of the unfortunate patient who lies in it, that excrementitious matter to eliminate which from the body nature had expressly appointed the disease?

My heart always sinks within me when I hear the good housewife, of every class, say, "I assure you the bed has been well slept

---

* I once told a "very good nurse" that the way in which her patient's room Nurses often was kept was quite enough to account for his sleeplessness; and she answered do not think quite good-humouredly she was not at all surprised at it—as if the state of the the sick-room room were, like the state of the weather, entirely out of her power. Now in what any business of sense was this woman to be called a "nurse?" theirs, but

† For the same reason if, after washing a patient, you must put the same only the sick. night-dress on him again, always give it a preliminary warm at the fire. The night-gown he has worn must be, to a certain extent, damp. It has now got cold from having been off him for a few minutes. The fire will dry and at the same time air it. This is much more important than with clean things.

in," and I can only hope it is not true. What? is the bed already saturated with somebody else's damp before my patient comes to exhale into it his own damp? Has it not had a single chance to be aired? No, not one. "It has been slept in every night."

The only way of really nursing a real patient is to have an *iron* bedstead, with rheocline springs, which are permeable by the air up to the very mattress (no vallance, of course), the mattress to be a thin hair one; the bed to be not above 3½ feet wide. If the patient be entirely confined to his bed, there should be *two* such bedsteads; each bed to be "made" with mattress, sheets, blankets, &c., complete —the patient to pass twelve hours in each bed; on no account to carry his sheets with him. The whole of the bedding to be hung up to air for each intermediate twelve hours. Of course there are many cases where this cannot be done at all—many more where only an approach to it can be made. I am indicating the ideal of nursing, and what I have actually had done. But about the kind of bedstead there can be no doubt, whether there be one or two provided.

There is a prejudice in favour of a wide bed—I believe it to be a prejudice. All the refreshment of moving a patient from one side to the other of his bed is far more effectually secured by putting him into a fresh bed; and a patient who is really very ill does not stray far in bed. But it is said there is no room to put a tray down on a narrow bed. No good nurse will ever put a tray on a bed at all. If the patient can turn on his side, he will eat more comfortably from a bed-side table; and on no account whatever should a bed ever be higher than a sofa. Otherwise the patient feels himself "out of humanity's reach"; he can get at nothing for himself: he can move nothing for himself. If the patient cannot turn, a table over the bed is a better thing. I need hardly say that a patient's bed should never have its side against the wall. The nurse must be able to get easily to both sides the bed, and to reach easily every part of the patient without stretching—a thing impossible if the bed be either too wide or too high.

When I see a patient in a room nine or ten feet high upon a bed between four and five feet high, with his head, when he is sitting up in bed, actually within two or three feet of the ceiling, I ask myself, is this expressly planned to produce that peculiarly distressing feeling common to the sick, viz., as if the walls and ceiling were closing in upon them, and they becoming sandwiches between floor and ceiling, which imagination is not, indeed, here so far from the truth? If, over and above this, the window stops short of the ceiling, then the patient's head may literally be raised above the stratum of fresh air, even when the window is open. Can human perversity any farther go, in unmaking the process of restoration which God has made? The fact is, that the heads of sleepers or of sick should never be higher than the throat of the chimney, which ensures their being in the current of best air. And we will not suppose it possible that you have closed your chimney with a chimney-board.

If a bed is higher than a sofa, the difference of the fatigue of getting in and out of bed will just make the difference. very often, to the patient (who can get in and out of bed at all) of being able to take a few minutes' exercise, either in the open air or in another room. It is so very odd that people never think of this, or of how many more times a patient who is in bed for the twenty-four hours is obliged to get in and out of bed than they are, who only, it is to be hoped, get into bed once and out of bed once during the twenty-four hours.

A patient's bed should always be in the lightest spot in the room; and he should be able to see out of window. *Nor in a dark place.*

I need scarcely say that the old four-post bed with curtains is utterly inadmissible, whether for sick or well. Hospital bedsteads are in many respects very much less objectionable than private ones. *Nor a four poster with curtains.*

There is reason to believe that not a few of the apparently unaccountable cases of scrofula among children proceed from the habit of sleeping with the head under the bed clothes, and so inhaling air already breathed, which is farther contaminated by exhalations from the skin. Patients are sometimes given to a similar habit, and it often happens that the bed clothes are so disposed that the patient must necessarily breathe air more or less contaminated by exhalations from his skin. A good nurse will be careful to attend to this. It is an important part, so to speak, of ventilation. *Scrofula often a result of disposition of bedclothes.*

It may be worth while to remark, that where there is any danger of bed-sores a blanket should never be placed *under* the patient. It retains damp and acts like a poultice. *Bed sores.*

Never use anything but light Witney blankets as bed covering for the sick. The heavy cotton impervious counterpane is bad, for the very reason that it keeps in the emanations from the sick person, while the blanket allows them to pass through. Weak patients are invariably distressed by a great weight of bed-clothes, which often prevents their getting any sound sleep whatever. *Heavy and impervious bed-clothes.*

NOTE.—One word about pillows. Every weak patient, be his illness what it may, suffers more or less from difficulty in breathing. To take the weight of the body off the poor chest, which is hardly up to its work as it is, ought therefore to be the object of the nurse in arranging his pillows. Now what does she do and what are the consequences? She piles the pillows one a-top of the other like a wall of bricks. The head is thrown upon the chest. And the shoulders are pushed forward, so as not to allow the lungs room to expand. The pillows, in fact, lean upon the patient, not the patient upon the pillows. It is impossible to give a rule for this, because it must vary with the figure of the patient. And tall patients suffer much more than short ones, because of the *drag* of the long limbs upon the waist. But the object is to support, with the pillows, the back *below* the breathing apparatus, to allow the shoulders room to fall back, and to support the head, without throwing it forward. The suffering of dying patients is immensely increased by neglect of these points. And many an invalid, too weak to drag about his pillows himself, slips his book or anything at hand behind the lower part of his back to support it.

IX. LIGHT.

It is the unqualified result of all my experience with the sick, that second only to their need of fresh air is their need of light; *Light essential to both health and recovery.*

that, after a close room, what hurts them most is a dark room.
And that it is not only light but direct sun-light they want. I had
rather have the power of carrying my patient about after the sun,
according to the aspect of the rooms, if circumstances permit, than
let him linger in a room when the sun is off. People think the effect
is upon the spirits only. This is by no means the case. The sun is
not only a painter but a sculptor. You admit that he does the
photograph. Without going into any scientific exposition we must
admit that light has quite as real and tangible effects upon the
human body. But this is not all. Who has not observed the
purifying effect of light, and especially of direct sunlight, upon the
air of a room? Here is an observation within everybody's experience. Go into a room where the shutters are always shut, (in a
sick room or a bedroom there should never be shutters shut), and
though the room be uninhabited, though the air has never been
polluted by the breathing of human beings, you will observe a close,
musty smell of corrupt air, of air *i. e.* unpurified by the effect of the
sun's rays. The mustiness of dark rooms and corners, indeed, is
proverbial. The cheerfulness of a room, the usefulness of light in
treating disease is all-important.

Aspect, view, and sunlight matters of first importance to the sick. A very high authority in hospital construction has said that
people do not enough consider the difference between wards and
dormitories in planning their buildings. But I go farther, and say,
that healthy people never remember the difference between *bed*-
rooms and *sick*-rooms, in making arrangements for the sick. To a
sleeper in health it does not signify what the view is from his bed.
He ought never to be in it excepting when asleep, and at night.
Aspect does not very much signify either (provided the sun reach
his bed-room some time in every day, to purify the air), because he
ought never to be in his bed-room except during the hours when
there is no sun. But the case is exactly reversed with the sick, even
should they be as many hours out of their beds as you are in yours,
which probably they are not. Therefore, that they should be able,
without raising themselves or turning in bed, to see out of window
from their beds, to see sky and sun-light at least, if you can show
them nothing else, I assert to be, if not of the very first importance
for recovery, at least something very near it. And you should therefore look to the position of the beds of your sick one of the very first
things. If they can see out of two windows instead of one, so much
the better. Again, the morning sun and the mid-day sun—the hours
when they are quite certain not to be up, are of more importance to
them, if a choice must be made, than the afternoon sun. Perhaps
you can take them out of bed in the afternoon and set them by the
window, where they can see the sun. But the best rule is, if
possible, to give them direct sun-light from the moment he rises till
the moment he sets.

Another great difference between the *bed*-room and the *sick*-room
is, that the *sleeper* has a very large balance of fresh air to begin with,
when he begins the night, if his room has been open all day as it
ought to be; the *sick* man has not, because all day he has been

breathing the air in the same room, and dirtying it by the emanations from himself. Far more care is therefore necessary to keep up a constant change of air in the sick room.

It is hardly necessary to add that there are acute cases, (particularly a few ophthalmic cases, and diseases where the eye is morbidly sensitive), where a subdued light is necessary. But a dark north room is inadmissible even for these. You can always moderate the light by blinds and curtains.

Heavy, thick, dark window or bed curtains should, however, hardly ever be used for any kind of sick in this country. A light white curtain at the head of the bed is, in general, all that is necessary, and a green blind to the window, to be drawn down only when necessary.

One of the greatest observers of human things (not physiological), says, in another language, " Where there is sun there is thought." All physiology goes to confirm this. Where is the shady side of deep valleys, there is cretinism. Where are cellars and the unsunned sides of narrow streets, there is the degeneracy and weakliness of the human race—mind and body equally degenerating. Put the pale withering plant and human being into the sun, and, if not too far gone, each will recover health and spirit. *Without sunlight, we degenerate body and mind.*

It is a curious thing to observe how almost all patients lie with their faces turned to the light, exactly as plants always make their way towards the light; a patient will even complain that it gives him pain " lying on that side." " Then why *do* you lie on that side ?" He does not know,—but we do. It is because it is the side towards the window. A fashionable physician has recently published in a government report that he always turns his patients' faces from the light. Yes, but nature is stronger than fashionable physicians, and depend upon it she turns the faces back and *towards* such light as she can get. Walk through the wards of a hospital, remember the bed sides of private patients you have seen, and count how many sick you ever saw lying with their faces towards the wall. *Almost all patients lie with their faces to the light.*

X. CLEANLINESS OF ROOMS AND WALLS.

It cannot be necessary to tell a nurse that she should be clean, or that she should keep her patient clean,—seeing that the greater part of nursing consists in preserving cleanliness. No ventilation can freshen a room or ward where the most scrupulous cleanliness is not observed. Unless the wind be blowing through the windows at the rate of twenty miles an hour, dusty carpets, dirty wainscots, musty curtains and furniture, will infallibly produce a close smell. I have lived in a large and expensively furnished London house, where the only constant inmate in two very lofty rooms, with opposite windows, was myself, and yet, owing to the abovementioned dirty circumstances, no opening of windows could ever keep those *Cleanliness of carpets and furniture.*

rooms free from closeness; but the carpet and curtains having been turned out of the rooms altogether, they became instantly as fresh as could be wished. It is pure nonsense to say that in London a room cannot be kept clean. Many of our hospitals show the exact reverse.

Dust never removed now. But no particle of dust is ever or can ever be removed or really got rid of by the present system of dusting. Dusting in these days means nothing but flapping the dust from one part of a room on to another with doors and windows closed. What you do it for I cannot think. You had much better leave the dust alone, if you are not going to take it away altogether. For from the time a room begins to be a room up to the time when it ceases to be one, no one atom of dust ever actually leaves its precincts. Tidying a room means nothing now but removing a thing from one place, which it has kept clean for itself, on to another and a dirtier one.* Flapping by way of cleaning is only admissible in the case of pictures, or anything made of paper. The only way I know to *remove* dust, the plague of all lovers of fresh air, is to wipe everything with a damp cloth. And all furniture ought to be so made as that it may be wiped with a damp cloth without injury to itself, and so polished as that it may be damped without injury to others. To dust, as it is now practised, truly means to distribute dust more equally over a room.

Floors. As to floors, the only really clean floor I know is the Berlin *lackered* floor, which is wet rubbed and dry rubbed every morning to remove the dust. The French *parquet* is always more or less dusty, although infinitely superior in point of cleanliness and healthiness to our absorbent floor.

For a sick room, a carpet is perhaps the worst expedient which could by any possibility have been invented. If you must have a carpet, the only safety is to take it up two or three times a year, instead of once. A dirty carpet literally infects the room. And if you consider the enormous quantity of organic matter from the feet of people coming in, which must saturate it, this is by no means surprising.

Papered, plastered, oil-painted walls. As for walls, the worst is the papered wall; the next worst is plaster. But the plaster can be redeemed by frequent lime-washing; the paper requires frequent renewing. A glazed paper gets rid of a

How a room is dusted. * If you like to clean your furniture by laying out your clean clothes upon your dirty chairs or sofa, this is one way certainly of doing it. Having witnessed the morning process called "tidying the room," for many years, and with ever-increasing astonishment, I can describe what it is. From the chairs, tables, or sofa, upon which the "things" have lain during the night, and which are therefore comparatively clean from dust or blacks, the poor "*things*" having "caught" it, they are removed to other chairs, tables, sofas, upon which you could write your name with your finger in the dust or blacks. The *other* side of the "things" is therefore now evenly dirtied or dusted. The housemaid then flaps every thing, or some things, not out of her reach, with a thing called a duster—the dust flies up, then re-settles more equally than it lay before the operation. The room has now been "put to rights."

good deal of the danger. But the ordinary bed-room paper is all that it ought *not* to be.*

The close connection between ventilation and cleanliness is shown in this. An ordinary light paper will last clean much longer if there is an Arnott's ventilator in the chimney than it otherwise would.

The best wall now extant is oil paint. From this you can wash the animal exuviæ.†

These are what make a room musty.

The best wall for a sick-room or ward that could be made is pure white non-absorbent cement or glass, or glazed tiles, if they were made sightly enough. *Best kind of wall for a sick-room.*

Air can be soiled just like water. If you blow into water you will soil it with the animal matter from your breath. So it is with air. Air is always soiled in a room where walls and carpets are saturated with animal exhalations.

Want of cleanliness, then, in rooms and wards, which you have to guard against, may arise in three ways.

1. Dirty air coming in from without, soiled by sewer emanations, the evaporation from dirty streets, smoke, bits of unburnt fuel, bits of straw, bits of horse dung. *Dirty air from without.*

If people would but cover the outside walls of their houses with plain or encaustic tiles, what an incalculable improvement would there be in light, cleanliness, dryness, warmth, and consequently economy. The play of a fire-engine would then effectually wash the outside of a house. This kind of *walling* would stand next to paving in improving the health of towns. *Best kind of wall for a house.*

2. Dirty air coming from within, from dust, which you often displace, but never remove. And this recalls what ought to be a *sine quâ non.* Have as few ledges in your room or ward as possible. And under no pretence have any ledge whatever out of sight. Dust accumulates there, and will never be wiped off. This is a certain way to soil the air. Besides this, the animal exhalations from your inmates saturate your furniture. And if you never clean your furniture properly, how can your rooms or wards be anything but musty? Ventilate as you please, the rooms will never be sweet. Besides this, there is a constant *degradation,* as it is called, taking place from everything except polished or glazed articles—*E. g.,* in colouring certain green papers arsenic is used. Now in the very dust even, which is lying about in rooms hung with this kind of green paper, arsenic has been distinctly detected. You see your dust is anything but harmless; yet you will let such dust lie about your ledges for months, your rooms for ever. *Dirty air from within.*

* I am sure that a person who has accustomed her senses to compare atmospheres proper and improper, for the sick and for children, could tell, blindfold, the difference of the air in old painted and in old papered rooms, *cæteris paribus.* The latter will always be musty, even with all the windows open. *Atmosphere in painted and papered rooms quite distinguishable.*

† If you like to wipe your dirty door, or some portion of your dirty wall, by hanging up your clean gown or shawl against it on a peg, this is one way certainly, and the most usual way, and generally the only way of cleaning either door or wall in a bed-room! *How to keep your wall clean at the expence of your clothes.*

Again, the fire fills the room with coal-dust.

Dirty air from the carpet.

3. Dirty air coming from the carpet. Above all, take care of the carpets, that the animal dirt left there by the feet of visitors does not stay there. Floors, unless the grain is filled up and polished, are just as bad. The smell from the floor of a school-room or ward, when any moisture brings out the organic matter by which it is saturated, might alone be enough to warn us of the mischief that is going on.

Remedies.

The outer air, then, can only be kept clean by sanitary improvements, and by consuming smoke. The expense in soap, which this single improvement would save, is quite incalculable.

The inside air can only be kept clean by excessive care in the ways mentioned above—to rid the walls, carpets, furniture, ledges, &c., of the organic matter and dust—dust consisting greatly of this organic matter—with which they become saturated, and which is what really makes the room musty.

Without cleanliness, you cannot have all the effect of ventilation; without ventilation, you can have no thorough cleanliness.

Very few people, be they of what class they may, have any idea of the exquisite cleanliness required in the sick-room. For much of what I have said applies less to the hospital than to the private sick-room. The smoky chimney, the dusty furniture, the utensils emptied but once a day, often keep the air of the sick constantly dirty in the best private houses.

The well have a curious habit of forgetting that what is to them but a trifling inconvenience, to be patiently " put up " with, is to the sick a source of suffering, delaying recovery, if not actually hastening death. The well are scarcely ever more than eight hours, at most, in the same room. Some change they can always make, if only for a few minutes. Even during the supposed eight hours, they can change their posture or their position in the room. But the sick man, who never leaves his bed, who cannot change by any movement of his own his air, or his light, or his warmth; who cannot obtain quiet, or get out of the smoke, or the smell, or the dust; he is really poisoned or depressed by what is to you the merest trifle.

" What can't be cured must be endured," is the very worst and most dangerous maxim for a nurse which ever was made. Patience and resignation in her are but other words for carelessness or indifference—contemptible, if in regard to herself; culpable, if in regard to her sick.

XI. PERSONAL CLEANLINESS.

Poisoning by the skin.

In almost all diseases, the function of the skin is, more or less, disordered; and in many most important diseases nature relieves herself almost entirely by the skin. This is particularly the case with children. But the excretion, which comes from the skin, is left there, unless removed by washing or by the clothes. Every nurse should keep this fact constantly in mind,—for, if she allow her sick to remain unwashed, or their clothing to remain on them after being saturated with perspiration or other excretion, she is interfering injuriously with the natural processes of health just as effectually as if she were to give the patient a dose of slow poison by the mouth. Poisoning by the skin is no less certain than poisoning by the mouth —only it is slower in its operation.

The amount of relief and comfort experienced by sick after the Ventilation skin has been carefully washed and dried, is one of the commonest and skin-cleanobservations made at a sick bed.　But it must not be forgotten that liness equally the comfort and relief so obtained are not all.　They are, in fact, essential. nothing more than a sign that the vital powers have been relieved by removing something that was oppressing them.　The nurse, therefore, must never put off attending to the personal cleanliness of her patient under the plea that all that is to be gained is a little relief, which can be quite as well given later.

In all well-regulated hospitals this ought to be, and generally is, attended to.　But it is very generally neglected with private sick.

Just as it is necessary to renew the air round a sick person frequently, to carry off morbid effluvia from the lungs and skin, by maintaining free ventilation, so is it necessary to keep the pores of the skin free from all obstructing excretions.　The object, both of ventilation and of skin-cleanliness, is pretty much the same,—to wit, removing noxious matter from the system as rapidly as possible.

Care should be taken in all these operations of sponging, washing, and cleansing the skin, not to expose too great a surface at once, so as to check the perspiration, which would renew the evil in another form.

The various ways of washing the sick need not here be specified, —the less so as the doctors ought to say which is to be used.

In several forms of diarrhœa, dysentery, &c., where the skin is hard and harsh, the relief afforded by washing with a great deal of soft soap is incalculable.　In other cases, sponging with tepid soap and water, then with tepid water and drying with a hot towel will be ordered.

Every nurse ought to be careful to wash her hands very frequently during the day.　If her face too, so much the better.

One word as to cleanliness merely as cleanliness.

Compare the dirtiness of the water in which you have washed Steaming and when it is cold without soap, cold with soap, hot with soap.　You rubbing the will find the first has hardly removed any dirt at all, the second a skin. little more, the third a great deal more.　But hold your hand over a cup of hot water for a minute or two, and then, by merely rubbing with the finger, you will bring off flakes of dirt or dirty skin.　After a vapour bath you may peel your whole self clean in this way.　What I mean is, that by simply washing or sponging with water you do not really clean your skin.　Take a rough towel, dip one corner in very hot water,—if a little spirit be added to it it will be more effectual,— and then rub as if you were rubbing the towel into your skin with your fingers.　The black flakes which will come off will convince

you that you were not clean before, however much soap and water
you have used. These flakes are what require removing. And you
can really keep yourself cleaner with a tumbler of hot water and a
rough towel and rubbing, than with a whole apparatus of bath and
soap and sponge, without rubbing. It is quite nonsense to say that
anybody need be dirty. Patients have been kept as clean by these
means on a long voyage, when a basin full of water could not be
afforded, and when they could not be moved out of their berths, as
if all the appurtenances of home had been at hand.

Washing, however, with a large quantity of water has quite other
effects than those of mere cleanliness. The skin absorbs the water
and becomes softer and more perspirable. To wash with soap and
soft water is, therefore, desirable from other points of view than that
of cleanliness.

XII. CHATTERING HOPES AND ADVICES.

Advising the
sick.

The sick man to his advisers.
"My advisers! Their name is legion.   *   *   *
Somehow or other, it seems a provision of the universal destinies,
that every man, woman, and child should consider him, her, or itself
privileged especially to advise me. Why? That is precisely what
I want to know." And this is what I have to say to them. I have
been advised to go to every place extant in and out of England—to
take every kind of exercise by every kind of cart, carriage—yes,
and even swing (!) and dumb-bell (!) in existence; to imbibe every
different kind of stimulus that ever has been invented. And this
when those *best* fitted to know, viz., medical men, after long and
close attendance, had declared any journey out of the question, had
prohibited any kind of motion whatever, had closely laid down the
diet and drink. What would my advisers say, were they the medical
attendants, and I the patient left their advice, and took the casual
adviser's? But the singularity in Legion's mind is this: it never
occurs to him that everybody else is doing the same thing, and that
I the patient *must* perforce say, in sheer self-defence, like Rosalind,
" I could not do with all."

Chattering
hopes the bane
of the sick.

"Chattering Hopes" may seem an odd heading. But I really
believe there is scarcely a greater worry which invalids have to endure
than the incurable hopes of their friends. There is no one practice
against which I can speak more strongly from actual personal experience, wide and long, of its effects during sickness observed both upon
others and upon myself. I would appeal most seriously to all friends,
visitors, and attendants of the sick to leave off this practice of
attempting to "cheer" the sick by making light of their danger and
by exaggerating their probabilities of recovery.

Far more now than formerly does the medical attendant tell the
truth to the sick who are really desirous to hear it about their own
state.

How intense is the folly, then, to say the least of it, of the friend, be he even a medical man, who thinks that his opinion, given after a cursory observation, will weigh with the patient, against the opinion of the medical attendant, given, perhaps, after years of observation, after using every help to diagnosis afforded by the stethoscope, the examination of pulse, tongue, &c. ; and certainly after much more observation than the friend can possibly have had.

Supposing the patient to be possessed of common sense,—how can the "favourable" opinion, if it is to be called an opinion at all, of the casual visitor "cheer " him,—when different from that of the experienced attendant? Unquestionably the latter may, and often does, turn out to be wrong. But which is most likely to be wrong?

The fact is, that the patient* is not "cheered " at all by these well-meaning, most tiresome friends. On the contrary, he is depressed and wearied. If, on the one hand, he exerts himself to tell each successive member of this too numerous conspiracy, whose name is legion, why he does not think as they do,—in what respect he is worse,—what symptoms exist that they know nothing of,—he is fatigued instead of " cheered," and his attention is fixed upon himself. In general, patients who are really ill, do not want to talk about themselves. Hypochondriacs do, but again I say we are not on the subject of hypochondriacs. *Patient does not want to talk of himself.*

If, on the other hand, and which is much more frequently the case, the patient says nothing, but the Shakespearian "Oh !" "Ah!" "Go to!" and " In good sooth!" in order to escape from the conversation about himself the sooner, he is depressed by want of sympathy. He feels isolated in the midst of friends. He feels what a convenience it would be, if there were any single person to whom he could speak simply and openly, without pulling the string upon himself of this *Absurd consolations put forth for the benefit of the sick.*

* There are, of course cases, as in first confinements, when an assurance from the doctor or experienced nurse to the frightened suffering woman that there is nothing unusual in her case, that she has nothing to fear but a few hours' pain, may cheer her most effectually. This is advice of quite another order. It is the advice of experience to utter inexperience. But the advice we have been referring to is the advice of inexperience to bitter experience; and, in general, amounts to nothing more than this, that *you* think *I* shall recover from consumption, because somebody knows somebody somewhere who has recovered from fever. *Absurd statistical comparisons made in common conversation by the most sensible people for the benefit of the sick.*

I have heard a doctor condemned whose patient did not, alas ! recover, because another doctor's patient of a *different* sex, of a *different* age, recovered from a *different* disease, in a *different* place. Yes, this is really true. If people who make these comparisons did but know (only they do not care to know), the care and preciseness with which such comparisons require to be made, (and are made), in order to be of any value whatever, they would spare their tongues. In comparing the deaths of one hospital with those of another, any statistics are justly considered absolutely valueless which do not give the ages, the sexes, and the diseases of all the cases. It does not seem necessary to mention this. It does not seem necessary to say that there can be no comparison between old men with dropsies and young women with consumptions. Yet the cleverest men and the cleverest women are often heard making such comparisons, ignoring entirely sex, age, disease, place—in fact, *all* the conditions essential to the question. It is the merest *gossip.*

shower-bath of silly hopes and encouragements; to whom he could express his wishes and directions without that person persisting in saying "I hope that it will please God yet to give you twenty years," or, "You have a long life of activity before you." How often we see at the end of biographies or of cases recorded in medical papers, "after a long illness A. died rather suddenly," or, "unexpectedly both to himself and to others." "Unexpectedly" to others, perhaps, who did not see, because they did not look; but by no means "unexpectedly to himself," as I feel entitled to believe, both from the internal evidence in such stories, and from watching similar cases: there was every reason to expect that A. would die, and he knew it; but he found it useless to insist upon his own knowledge to his friends.

In these remarks I am alluding neither to acute cases which terminate rapidly nor to "nervous" cases.

By the first much interest in their own danger is very rarely felt. In writings of fiction, whether novels or biographies, these death-beds are generally depicted as almost seraphic in lucidity of intelligence. Sadly large has been my experience in death-beds, and I can only say that I have seldom or never seen such. Indifference, excepting with regard to bodily suffering, or to some duty the dying man desires to perform, is the far more usual state.

The "nervous case," on the other hand, delights in figuring to himself and others a fictitious danger.

But the long chronic case, who knows too well himself, and who has been told by his physician that he will never enter active life again, who feels that every month he has to give up something he could do the month before—oh! spare such sufferers your chattering hopes. You do not know how you worry and weary them. Such real sufferers cannot bear to talk of themselves, still less to hope for what they cannot at all expect.

So also as to all the advice showered so profusely upon such sick, to leave off some occupation, to try some other doctor, some other house, climate, pill, powder, or specific; I say nothing of the inconsistency—for these advisers are sure to be the same persons who exhorted the sick man not to believe his own doctor's prognostics, because "doctors are always mistaken," but to believe some other doctor, because "this doctor is always right." Sure also are these advisers to be the persons to bring the sick man fresh occupation, while exhorting him to leave his own.

Wonderful presumption of the advisers of the sick. Wonderful is the face with which friends, lay and medical, will come in and worry the patient with recommendations to do something or other, having just as little knowledge as to its being feasible, or even safe for him, as if they were to recommend a man to take exercise, not knowing he had broken his leg. What would the friend say, if *he* were the medical attendant, and if the patient, because some *other* friend had come in, because somebody, anybody, nobody, had recommended something, anything, nothing, were to disregard *his* orders, and take that other body's recommendation? But people never think of this.

A celebrated historical personage has related the common- Advisers the
places which, when on the eve of executing a remarkable reso- same now as
lution, were showered in nearly the same words by every one two hundred
years ago.
around successively for a period of six months. To these the
personage states that it was found least trouble always to reply
the same thing, viz., that it could not be supposed that such a
resolution had been taken without sufficient previous consideration.
To patients enduring every day for years from every friend or
acquaintance, either by letter or *vivâ voce*, some torment of this kind,
I would suggest the same answer. It would indeed be spared,
if such friends and acquaintances would but consider for one
moment, that it is probable the patient has heard such advice at
least fifty times before, and that, had it been practicable, it would
have been practised long ago. But of such consideration there
appears to be no chance. Strange, though true, that people should
be just the same in these things as they were a few hundred years
ago!

To me these commonplaces, leaving their smear upon the cheerful,
single-hearted, constant devotion to duty, which is so often seen in
the decline of such sufferers, recall the slimy trail left by the snail on
the sunny southern garden-wall loaded with fruit.

No mockery in the world is so hollow as the advice showered Mockery of
the advice
given to sick.
upon the sick. It is of no use for the sick to say anything, for what
the adviser wants is, *not* to know the truth about the state of the
patient, but to turn whatever the sick may say to the support of his
own argument, set forth, it must be repeated, without any inquiry
whatever into the patient's real condition. "But it would be impertinent or indecent in me to make such an inquiry," says the
adviser. True; and how much more impertinent is it to give your
advice when you can know nothing about the truth, and admit you
could not inquire into it.

To nurses I say—these are the visitors who do your patient
harm. When you hear him told:—1. That he has nothing the
matter with him, and that he wants cheering. 2. That he is com-
mitting suicide, and that he wants preventing. 3. That he is the
tool of somebody who makes use of him for a purpose. 4. That he
will listen to nobody, but is obstinately bent upon his own way;
and 5. That he ought to be called to the sense of duty, and is flying
in the face of Providence;—then know that your patient is receiving
all the injury that he can receive from a visitor.

How little the real sufferings of illness are known or understood.
How little does any one in good health fancy him or even *her*self into
the life of a sick person.

Do, you who are about the sick or who visit the sick, try and give Means of
them pleasure, remember to tell them what will do so. How often in giving plea-
such visits the sick person has to do the whole conversation, exerting sure to the
sick.
his own imagination and memory, while you would take the visitor,
absorbed in his own anxieties, making no effort of memory or
imagination, for the sick person. "Oh! my dear, I have so much to
think of, I really quite forgot to tell him that; besides, I thought he

would know it," says the visitor to another friend. How could "he know it"? Depend upon it, the people who say this are really those who have little "to think of." There are many burthened with business who always manage to keep a pigeon-hole in their minds, full of things to tell the "invalid."

I do not say, don't tell him your anxieties—I believe it is good for him and good for you too; but if you tell him what is anxious, surely you can remember to tell him what is pleasant too.

A sick person does so enjoy hearing good news:—for instance, of a love and courtship, while in progress to a good ending. If you tell him only when the marriage takes place, he loses half the pleasure, which God knows he has little enough of; and ten to one but you have told him of some love-making with a bad ending.

A sick person also intensely enjoys hearing of any *material* good, any positive or practical success of the right. He has so much of books and fiction, of principles, and precepts, and theories; do, instead of advising him with advice he has heard at least fifty times before, tell him of one benevolent act which has really succeeded practically,—it is like a day's health to him.*

You have no idea what the craving of sick with undiminished power of thinking, but little power of doing, is to hear of good practical action, when they can no longer partake in it.

Do observe these things with the sick. Do remember how their life is to them disappointed and incomplete. You see them lying there with miserable disappointments, from which they can have no escape but death, and you can't remember to tell them of what would give them so much pleasure, or at least an hour's variety.

They don't want you to be lachrymose and whining with them, they like you to be fresh and active and interested, but they cannot bear absence of mind, and they are so tired of the advice and preaching they receive from every body, no matter whom it is, they see.

There is no better society than babies and sick people for one another. Of course you must manage this so that neither shall suffer from it, which is perfectly possible. If you think the "air of the sick room" bad for the baby, why it is bad for the invalid too, and, therefore, you will of course correct it for both. It freshens up a sick person's whole mental atmosphere to see "the baby." And a very young child, if unspoiled, will generally adapt itself wonderfully to the ways of a sick person, if the time they spend together is not too long.

If you knew how unreasonably sick people suffer from reasonable causes of distress, you would take more pains about all these things. An infant laid upon the sick bed will do the sick person, thus suffering, more good than all your logic. A piece of good news will do the same. Perhaps you are afraid of "disturbing" him. You say there is no comfort for his present cause of affliction. It is perfectly

---

* A small pet animal is often an excellent companion for the sick, for long chronic cases especially. A pet bird in a cage is sometimes the only pleasure of an invalid confined for years to the same room. If he can feed and clean the animal himself, he ought always to be encouraged to do so.

reasonable. The distinction is this, if he is obliged to act, do not "disturb" him with another subject of thought just yet; help him to do what he wants to do: but, if he *has* done this, or if nothing *can* be done, then "disturb" him by all means. You will relieve, more effectually, unreasonable suffering from reasonable causes by telling him "the news," showing him "the baby," or giving him something new to think of or to look at than by all the logic in the world.

It has been very justly said that the sick are like children in this, that there is no *proportion* in events to them. Now it is your business as their visitor to restore this right proportion for them—to shew them what the rest of the world is doing. How can they find it out otherwise? You will find them far more open to conviction than children in this. And you will find that their unreasonable intensity of suffering from unkindness, from want of sympathy, &c., will disappear with their freshened interest in the big world's events. But then you must be able to give them real interests, not gossip.

NOTE.—There are two classes of patients which are unfortunately becoming more common every day, especially among women of the richer orders, to whom all these remarks are pre-eminently inapplicable. 1. Those who make health an excuse for doing nothing, and at the same time allege that the being able to do nothing is their only grief. 2. Those who have brought upon themselves ill-health by over pursuit of amusement, which they and their friends have most unhappily called intellectual activity. I scarcely know a greater injury that can be inflicted than the advice too often given to the first class "to vegetate"— or than the admiration too often bestowed on the latter class for "pluck." *Two new classes of patients peculiar to this generation.*

XIII. OBSERVATION OF THE SICK.

There is no more silly or universal question scarcely asked than this, "Is he better?" Ask it of the medical attendant, if you please. But of whom else, if you wish for a real answer to your question, would you ask it? Certainly not of the casual visitor; certainly not of the nurse, while the nurse's observation is so little exercised as it is now. What you want are facts, not opinions—for who can have any opinion of any value as to whether the patient is better or worse, excepting the constant medical attendant, or the really observing nurse? *What is the use of the question, Is he better?*

The most important practical lesson that can be given to nurses is to teach them what to observe—how to observe—what symptoms indicate improvement—what the reverse—which are of importance —which are of none—which are the evidence of neglect—and of what kind of neglect.

All this is what ought to make part, and an essential part, of the training of every nurse. At present how few there are, either professional or unprofessional, who really know at all whether any sick person they may be with is better or worse.

The vagueness and looseness of the information one receives in answer to that much abused question, "Is he better?" would be ludicrous, if it were not painful. The only sensible answer (in the present state of knowledge about sickness) would be "How can I know? I cannot tell how he was when I was not with him."

I can record but a very few specimens of the answers* which I have heard made by friends and nurses, and accepted by physicians and surgeons at the very bed-side of the patient, who could have contradicted every word, but did not—sometimes from amiability, often from shyness, oftenest from languor!

"How often have the bowels acted, nurse?" "Once, sir." This generally means that the utensil has been emptied once, it having been used perhaps seven or eight times.

"Do you think the patient is much weaker than he was six weeks ago?" "Oh no, sir; you know it is very long since he has been up and dressed, and he can get across the room now." This means that the nurse has not observed that whereas six weeks ago he sat up and occupied himself in bed, he now lies still doing nothing; that, although he can "get across the room," he cannot stand for five seconds.

Another patient who is eating well, recovering steadily, although slowly, from fever, but cannot walk or stand, is represented to the doctor as making no progress at all.

---

* It is a much more difficult thing to speak the truth than people commonly imagine. There is the want of observation *simple*, and the want of observation *compound*, compounded, that is, with the imaginative faculty. Both may equally intend to speak the truth. The information of the first is simply defective. That of the second is much more dangerous. The first gives, in answer to a question asked about a thing that has been before his eyes perhaps for years, information exceedingly imperfect, or says, he does not know. He has never observed. And people simply think him stupid.

The second has observed just as little, but imagination immediately steps in, and he describes the whole thing from imagination merely, being perfectly convinced all the while that he has seen or heard it; or he will repeat a whole conversation, as if it were information which had been addressed to him ; whereas it is merely what he has himself said to somebody else. This is the commonest of all. These people do not even observe that they have *not* observed nor remember that they have forgotten.

Courts of justice seem to think that any body can speak "the whole truth and nothing but the truth," if he does but intend it. It requires many faculties combined of observation and memory to speak "the whole truth" and to say "nothing but the truth."

"I knows I fibs dreadful : but believe me, Miss, I never finds out I have fibbed until they tells me so," was a remark actually made. It is also one of much more extended application than most people have the least idea of.

Concurrence of testimony, which is so often adduced as final proof, may prove nothing more, as is well known to those accustomed to deal with the unobservant imaginative, than that one person has told his story a great many times

I have heard thirteen persons "concur" in declaring that a fourteenth, who had never left his bed, went to a distant chapel every morning at seven o'clock.

I have heard persons in perfect good faith declare, that a man came to dine every day at the house where they lived, who had never dined there once ; that a person had never taken the sacrament, by whose side they had twice at least knelt at Communion; that but one meal a day came out of a hospital kitchen, which for six weeks they had seen provide from three to five and six meals a day. Such instances might be multiplied *ad infinitum* if necessary.

Questions, too, as asked now (but too generally) of or about Leading ques-
patients, would obtain no information at all about them, even if the tions useless
person asked of had every information to give. The question is or misleading.
generally a leading question; and it is singular that people never
think what must be the answer to this question before they ask
it: for instance, " Has he had a good night?" Now, one patient
will think he has a bad night if he has not slept ten hours without
waking. Another does not think he has a bad night if he has had
intervals of dosing occasionally. The same answer has actually been
given as regarded two patients—one who had been entirely sleepless
for five times twenty-four hours, and died of it, and another who had
not slept the sleep of a regular night, without waking. Why cannot
the question be asked, How many hours' sleep has —— had? and
at what hours of the night?* " I have never closed my eyes all
night," an answer as frequently made when the speaker has had
several hours' sleep as when he has had none, would then be less
often said. Lies, intentional and unintentional, are much seldomer
told in answer to precise than to leading questions. Another
frequent error is to inquire whether one cause remains, and not
whether the effect which may be produced by a great many different
causes, *not* inquired after, remains. As when it is asked, whether
there was noise in the street last night; and if there were not, the
patient is reported, without more ado, to have had a good night.
Patients are completely taken aback by these kinds of leading questions, and give only the exact amount of information asked for, even
when they know it to be completely misleading. The shyness of
patients is seldom allowed for.

How few there are who, by five or six pointed questions, can
elicit the whole case and get accurately to know and to be able to
report *where* the patient is.

I knew a very clever physician, of large dispensary and hospital Means of
practice, who invariably began his examination of each patient with obtaining
" Put your finger where you be bad." That man would never waste inaccurate
his time with collecting inaccurate information from nurse or patient. information.
Leading questions always collect inaccurate information.

At a recent celebrated trial, the following leading question was
put successively to nine distinguished medical men. " Can you attribute these symptoms to anything else but poison?" And out of the
nine, eight answered " No!" without any qualification whatever. It
appeared, upon cross-examination :—1. That none of them had ever
seen a case of the kind of poisoning supposed. 2. That none of them
had ever seen a case of the kind of disease to which the death, if not
to poison, was attributable. 3. That none of them were even aware

---

* This is important, because on this depends what the remedy will be. If a
patient sleeps two or three hours early in the night, and then does not sleep
again at all, ten to one it is not a narcotic he wants, but food or stimulus, or
perhaps only warmth. If on the other hand, he is restless and awake all night,
and is drowsy in the morning, he probably wants sedatives, either quiet, coolness,
or medicine, a lighter diet, or all four. Now the doctor should be told this, or
how can he judge what to give?

of the main fact of the disease and condition to which the death was attributable.

Surely nothing stronger can be adduced to prove what use leading questions are of, and what they lead to.

I had rather not say how many instances I have known, where, owing to this system of leading questions, the patient has died, and the attendants have been actually unaware of the principal feature of the case.

As to food patient takes or does not take.
It is useless to go through all the particulars, besides sleep, in which people have a peculiar talent for gleaning inaccurate information. As to food, for instance, I often think that most common question, How is your appetite? can only be put because the questioner believes the questioned has really nothing the matter with him, which is very often the case. But where there is, the remark holds good which has been made about sleep. The *same* answer will often be made as regards a patient who cannot take two ounces of solid food per diem, and a patient who does not enjoy five meals a day as much as usual.

Again, the question, How is your appetite? is often put when How is your digestion? is the question meant. No doubt the two things depend on one another. But they are quite different. Many a patient can eat, if you can only "tempt his appetite." The fault lies in your not having got him the thing that he fancies. But many another patient does not care between grapes and turnips,— everything is equally distasteful to him. He would try to eat anything which would do him good; but everything "makes him worse." The fault here generally lies in the cooking. It is not his "appetite" which requires "tempting," it is his digestion which requires sparing. And good sick cookery will save the digestion half its work.

There may be four different causes, any one of which will produce the same result, viz., the patient slowly starving to death from want of nutrition:

1. Defect in cooking;
2. Defect in choice of diet;
3. Defect in choice of hours for taking diet;
4. Defect of appetite in patient.

Yet, all these are generally comprehended in the one sweeping assertion that the patient has "no appetite."

Surely many lives might be saved by drawing a closer distinction; for the remedies are as diverse as the causes. The remedy for the first is, to cook better; for the second, to choose other articles of diet; for the third, to watch for the hours when the patient is in want of food; for the fourth, to show him what he likes, and sometimes unexpectedly. But no one of these remedies will do for any other of the defects not corresponding with it.

I cannot too often repeat that patients are generally either too languid to observe these things, or too shy to speak about them; nor is it well that they should be made to observe them, it fixes their attention upon themselves.

Again, I say, what *is* the nurse or friend there for except to take note of these things, instead of the patient doing so?*

Again, the question is sometimes put, Is there diarrhœa? And the answer will be the same, whether it is just merging into cholera, whether it is a trifling degree brought on by some trifling indiscretion, which will cease the moment the cause is removed, or whether there is no diarrhœa at all, but simply relaxed bowels. *As to diarrhœa.*

It is useless to multiply instances of this kind. As long as observation is so little cultivated as it is now, I do believe that it is better for the physician *not* to see the friends of the patient at all. They will oftener mislead him than not. And as often by making the patient out worse as better than he really is.

In the case of infants, *everything* must depend upon the accurate observation of the nurse or mother who has to report. And how seldom is this condition of accuracy fulfilled.

A celebrated man, though celebrated only for foolish things, has told us that one of his main objects in the education of his son, was to give him a ready habit of accurate observation, a certainty of perception, and that for this purpose one of his means was a month's course as follows:—he took the boy rapidly past a toy-shop; the father and son then described to each other as many of the objects as they could, which they had seen in passing the windows, noting them down with pencil and paper, and returning afterwards to verify their own accuracy. The boy always succeeded best, *e.g.*, if the father described 30 objects, the boy did 40, and scarcely ever made a mistake. *Means of cultivating sound and ready observation.*

I have often thought how wise a piece of education this would be for much higher objects ; and in our calling of nurses the thing itself is essential. For it may safely be said, not that the habit of ready and correct observation will by itself make us useful nurses, but that without it we shall be useless with all our devotion.

I have known a nurse in charge of a set of wards who not only carried in her head all the little varieties in the diets which each patient was allowed to fix for himself, but also exactly what each patient had taken during each day. I have known another nurse in charge of one single patient, who took away his meals day after day all but untouched, and never knew it.

If you find it helps you to note down such things on a bit of paper, in pencil, by all means do so. I think it more often lames than strengthens the memory and observation. But if you cannot get the habit of observation one way or other, you had better give up the being a nurse, for it is not your calling, however kind and anxious you may be.

* It is commonly supposed that the nurse is there to spare the patient from making physical exertion for himself—I would rather say that she ought to be there to spare him from taking thought for himself. And I am quite sure, that if the patient were spared all thought for himself, and *not* spared all physical exertion, he would be infinitely the gainer. The reverse is generally the case in the private house. In the hospital it is the relief from all anxiety, afforded by the rules of a well-regulated institution, which has often such a beneficial effect upon the patient. *More important to spare the patient thought than physical exertion.*

Surely you can learn at least to judge with the eye how much an oz. of solid food is, how much an oz. of liquid. You will find this helps your observation and memory very much, you will then say to yourself "A. took about an oz. of his meat to day;" "B. took three times in 24 hours about ¼ pint of beef tea;" instead of saying "B. has taken nothing all day," or "I gave A. his dinner as usual."

Sound and ready observation essential in a nurse.

I have known several of our real old-fashioned hospital "sisters," who could, as accurately as a measuring glass, measure out all their patients' wine and medicine by the eye, and never be wrong. I do not recommend this, one must be very sure of one's self to do it. I only mention it, because if a nurse can by practice measure medicine by the eye, surely she is no nurse who cannot measure by the eye about how much food (in oz.) her patient has taken.* In hospitals those who cut up the diets give with quite sufficient accuracy, to each patient, his 12 oz. or his 6 oz. of meat without weighing. Yet a nurse will often have patients loathing all food and incapable of any will to get well, who just tumble over the contents of the plate or dip the spoon in the cup to deceive the nurse, and she will take it away without ever seeing that there is just the same quantity of food as when she brought it, and she will tell the doctor, too, that the patient

English women have great capacity of but little practice in close observation.

* It may be too broad an assertion, and it certainly sounds like a paradox. But I think that in no country are women to be found so deficient in ready and sound observation as in England, while peculiarly capable of being trained to it. The French or Irish woman is too quick of perception to be so sound an observer— the Teuton is too slow to be so ready an observer as the English woman might be. Yet English women lay themselves open to the charge so often made against them by men, viz., that they are not to be trusted in handicrafts to which their strength is quite equal, for want of a practised and steady observation. In countries where women (with average intelligence certainly not superior to that of Englishwomen) are employed, e. g., in dispensing, men responsible for what these women do (not theorizing about man's and woman's "missions"), have stated that they preferred the service of women to that of men, as being more exact, more careful, and incurring fewer mistakes of inadvertence.

Now certainly Englishwomen are peculiarly capable of attaining to this.

I remember when a child, hearing the story of an accident, related by some one who sent two girls to fetch a "bottle of salvolatile from her room;" "Mary could not stir," she said, "Fanny ran and fetched a bottle that was not salvolatile, and that was not in my room."

Now this sort of thing pursues every one through life. A woman is asked to fetch a large new bound red book, lying on the table by the window, and she fetches five small old bound brown books lying on the shelf by the fire. And this, though she has "put that room to rights" every day for a month perhaps, and must have observed the books every day, lying in the same places, for a month, if she had any observation.

Habitual observation is the more necessary, when any sudden call arises. If "Fanny" had observed "the bottle of salvolatile" in "the aunt's room," every day she was there, she would more probably have found it when it was suddenly wanted.

ı There are two causes for these mistakes of inadvertence. 1. A want of ready attention; only part of the request is heard at all. 2. A want of the habit of observation.

To a nurse I would add, take care that you always put the same things in the same places; you don't know how suddenly you may be called on some day to find something, and may not be able to remember in your haste where you your-self had put it, if your memory is not in the habit of seeing the thing there always.

has eaten all his diets as usual, when all she ought to have meant is that she has taken away his diets as usual.

Now what kind of a nurse is this?

I would call attention to something else, in which nurses fre- Difference of quently fail in observation.   There is a well-marked distinction excitable and between the excitable and what I will call the *accumulative* tempera- *accumulative* ment in patients.   One will blaze up at once, under any shock or $\frac{tempera-}{ments.}$ anxiety, and sleep very comfortably after it; another will seem quite calm and even torpid, under the same shock, and people say, "He hardly felt it at all," yet you will find him some time after slowly sinking.   The same remark applies to the action of narcotics, of ape- rients, which, in the one, take effect directly, in the other not perhaps for twenty-four hours.   A journey, a visit, an unwonted exertion, will affect the one immediately, but he recovers after it; the other bears it very well at the time, apparently, and dies or is pros- trated for life by it.   People often say how difficult the excitable temperament is to manage.   I say how difficult is the *accumulative* temperament.   With the first you have an out-break which you could anticipate, and it is all over.   With the second you never know where you are—you never know when the consequences are over.   And it requires your closest observation to know what *are* the consequences of what—for the consequent by no means follows immediately upon the antecedent—and coarse observation is utterly at fault.

Almost all superstitions are owing to bad observation, to the *post* Superstition *hoc, ergo propter hoc ;* and bad observers are almost all superstitious. the fruit of Farmers used to attribute disease among cattle to witchcraft; wed- bad observa- dings have been attributed to seeing one magpie, deaths to seeing tion. three; and I have heard the most highly educated now-a-days draw consequences for the sick closely resembling these.

Another remark: although there is unquestionably a physi- Physiog- ognomy of disease as well as of health; of all parts of the body, the nomy of disease face is perhaps the one which tells the least to the common observer little shewn or the casual visitor.   Because, of all parts of the body, it is by the face. the one most exposed to other influences, besides health.   And people never, or scarcely ever, observe enough to know how to dis- tinguish between the effect of exposure, of robust health, of a tender skin, of a tendency to congestion, of suffusion, flushing, or many other things.   Again, the face is often the last to shew emaciation. I should say that the hand was a much surer test than the face, both as to flesh, colour, circulation, &c., &c.   It is true that there are *some* diseases which are only betrayed at all by something in the face, *e.g.*, the eye or the tongue, as great irritability of brain by the appearance of the pupil of the eye.   But we are talking of casual, not minute, observation.   And few minute observers will hesitate to say that far more untruth than truth is conveyed by the oft repeated words, He *looks* well, or ill, or better or worse.

Wonderful is the way in which people will go upon the slightest observation, or often upon no observation at all, or upon some *saw* which the world's experience, if it had any, would have pronounced utterly false long ago.

F

I have known patients dying of sheer pain, exhaustion, and want of sleep, from one of the most lingering and painful diseases known, preserve, till within a few days of death, not only the healthy colour of the cheek, but the mottled appearance of a robust child. And scores of times have I heard these unfortunate creatures assailed with, "I am glad to see you looking so well." "I see no reason why you should not live till ninety years of age." "Why don't you take a little more exercise and amusement?" with all the other commonplaces with which we are so familiar.

There is, unquestionably, a physiognomy of disease. Let the nurse learn it.

The experienced nurse can always tell that a person has taken a narcotic the night before by the patchiness of the colour about the face, when the re-action of depression has set in; that very colour which the inexperienced will point to as a proof of health.

There is, again, a faintness, which does not betray itself by the colour at all, or in which the patient becomes brown instead of white. There is a faintness of another kind which, it is true, can always be seen by the paleness.

But the nurse seldom distinguishes. She will talk to the patient who is too faint to move, without the least scruple, unless he is pale and unless, luckily for him, the muscles of the throat are affected and he loses his voice.

Yet these two faintnesses are perfectly distinguishable, by the mere countenance of the patient.

Peculiarities of patients.

Again, the nurse must distinguish between the idiosyncracies or patients. One likes to suffer out all his suffering alone, to be as little looked after as possible. Another likes to be perpetually made much of and pitied, and to have some one always by him. Both these peculiarities might be observed and indulged much more than they are. For quite as often does it happen that a busy attendance is forced upon the first patient, who wishes for nothing but to be "let alone," as that the second is left to think himself neglected.

Nurse must observe for herself increase of patient's weakness, patient will not tell her.

Again, I think that few things press so heavily on one suffering from long and incurable illness, as the necessity of recording in words from time to time, for the information of the nurse, who will not otherwise see, that he cannot do this or that, which he could do a month or a year ago. What is a nurse there for if she cannot observe these things for herself? Yet I have known—and known too among those—and *chiefly* among those—whom money and position put in possession of everything which money and position could give—I have known, I say, more accidents, (fatal, slowly or rapidly,) arising from this want of observation among nurses than from almost anything else. Because a patient could get out of a warm-bath alone a month ago—because a patient could walk as far as his bell a week ago, the nurse concludes that he can do so now. She has never observed the change; and the patient is lost from being left in a helpless state of exhaustion, till some one accidentally comes in. And this not from any unexpected apoplectic, paralytic, or fainting fit (though even these could be expected far more, at least, than they are now, if we did but *observe*). No, from the expected, or to be expected, inevitable, visible, calculable, uninterrupted increase of weakness, which none need fail to observe.

Again, a patient not usually confined to bed, is compelled by an attack of diarrhœa, vomiting, or other accident, to keep his bed for a few days; he gets up for the first time, and the nurse lets him go into another room, without coming in, a few minutes afterwards, to look after him. It never occurs to her that he is quite certain to be faint, or cold, or to want something. She says, as her excuse, Oh, he does not like to be fidgetted after. Yes, he said so some weeks ago; but he never said he did not like to be "fidgetted after," when he is in the state he is in now; and if he did, you ought to make some excuse to go in to him. More patients have been lost in this way than is at all generally known, viz., from relapses brought on by being left for an hour or two faint, or cold, or hungry, after getting up for the first time. *(margin: Accidents arising from the nurse's want of observation.)*

Yet it appears that scarcely any improvement in the faculty of observing is being made. Vast has been the increase of knowledge in pathology—that science which teaches us the final change produced by disease on the human frame—scarce any in the art of observing the signs of the change while in progress. Or, rather, is it not to be feared that observation, as an essential part of medicine, has been declining? *(margin: Is the faculty of observing on the decline.)*

Which of us has not heard fifty times, from one or another, a nurse, or a friend of the sick, aye, and a medical friend too, the following remark:—"So A is worse, or B is dead. I saw him the day before; I thought him so much better; there certainly was no appearance from which one could have expected so sudden (?) a change." I have never heard any one say, though one would think it the more natural thing, "There *must* have been *some* appearance, which I should have seen if I had but looked; let me try and remember what there was, that I may observe another time." No, this is not what people say. They boldly assert that there was nothing to observe, not that their observation was at fault.

Let people who have to observe sickness and death look back and try to register in their observation the appearances which have preceded relapse, attack, or death, and not assert that there were none, or that there were not the *right* ones.*

A want of the habit of observing conditions and an inveterate habit of taking averages are each of them often equally misleading. *(margin: Observation of general conditions.)*

* It falls to few ever to have had the opportunity of observing the different aspects which the human face puts on at the sudden approach of certain forms of death by violence; and as it is a knowledge of little use I only mention it here as being the most startling example of what I mean. In the nervous temperament the face becomes pale (this is the only *recognized* effect); in the sanguine temperament purple; in the bilious yellow, or every manner of colour in patches. Now, it is generally supposed that paleness is the one indication of almost any violent change in the human being, whether from terror, disease, or anything else. There can be no more false observation. Granted, it is the one recognized livery, as I have said—*de rigueur* in novels, but nowhere else. *(margin: Approach of death, paleness by no means an invariable effect, as we find in novels.)*

Men whose profession like that of medical men leads them to observe only, or chiefly, palpable and permanent organic changes are often just as wrong in their opinion of the result as those who do not observe at all. For instance, there is a broken leg; the surgeon has only to look at it once to know; it will not be different if he sees it in the morning to what it would have been had he seen it in the evening. And in whatever conditions the patient is, or is likely to be, there will still be the broken leg, until it is set. The same with many organic diseases. An experienced physician has but to feel the pulse once, and he knows that there is aneurism which will kill some time or other.

But with the great majority of cases, there is nothing of the kind; and the power of forming any correct opinion as to the result must entirely depend upon an enquiry into all the conditions in which the patient lives. In a complicated state of society in large towns, death, as every one of great experience knows, is far less often produced by any one organic disease than by some illness, after many other diseases, producing just the sum of exhaustion necessary for death. There is nothing so absurd, nothing so misleading as the verdict one so often hears: So-and-so has no organic disease,—there is no reason why he should not live to extreme old age; sometimes the clause is added, sometimes not: Provided he has quiet, good food, good air, &c., &c., &c.; the verdict is repeated by ignorant people *without* the latter clause; or there is no possibility of the conditions of the latter clause being obtained; and this, the *only* essential part of the whole, is made of no effect. I have heard a physician, deservedly eminent, assure the friends of a patient of his recovery. Why? Because he had now prescribed a course, every detail of which the patient had followed for years. And because he had forbidden a course which the patient could not by any possibility alter.*

* I have known two cases, the one of a man who intentionally and repeatedly displaced a dislocation, and was kept and petted by all the surgeons, the other of one who was pronounced to have nothing the matter with him, there being no organic change perceptible, but who died within the week. In both these cases, it was the nurse who, by accurately pointing out what she had accurately observed, to the doctors, saved the one case from persevering in a fraud, the other from being discharged when actually in a dying state.

I will even go further and say, that in diseases which have their origin in the feeble or irregular action of some function, and not in organic change, it is quite an accident if the doctor who sees the case only once a day, and generally at the same time, can form any but a negative idea of its real condition. In the middle of the day, when such a patient has been refreshed by light and air, by his tea, his beef tea, and his brandy, by hot bottles to his feet, by being washed and by clean linen, you can scarcely believe that he is the same person as lay with a rapid fluttering pulse, with puffed eye-lids, with short breath, cold limbs, and unsteady hands, this morning. Now what is a nurse to do in such a case? Not cry, "Lord bless you, sir, why you'd have thought he were a dying all night." This may be true, but it is not the way to impress with the truth a doctor, more capable of forming a judgment from the facts, if he did but know them, than you are. What he wants is not your opinion, however respectfully given, but your facts. In all diseases it is important, but in diseases which do not run a distinct and fixed course, it is not only important, it is essential that the facts the nurse alone can observe, should be accurately observed, and accurately reported to the doctor.

Undoubtedly a person of no scientific knowledge whatever but of observation and experience in these kinds of conditions, will be able to arrive at a much truer guess as to the probable duration of life of members of a family or inmates of a house, than the most scientific physician to whom the same persons are brought to have their pulse felt; no enquiry being made into their conditions.

In Life Insurance and such like societies, were they instead of having the persons examined by a medical man, to have the houses, conditions, ways of life, of these persons examined, at how much truer results would they arrive! W. Smith appears a fine hale man, but it might be known that the next cholera epidemic he runs a bad chance. Mr. and Mrs. J. are a strong healthy couple, but it might be known that they live in such a house, in such a part of London, so near the river that they will kill four-fifths of their children ; which of the children will be the ones to survive might also be known.

Averages again seduce us away from minute observation. "Average mortalities" merely tell that so many per cent. die in this town and so many in that, per annum. But whether A or B will be among these, the "average rate" of course does not tell. We know, say, that from 22 to 24 per 1,000 will die in London next year. But minute enquiries into conditions enable us to know that in such a district, nay, in such a street,—or even on one side of that street, in such a particular house, or even on one floor of that particular *"Average rate of mortality" tells us only that so many per cent. will die. Observation must tell us which in the hundred they will be who will die.*

I must direct the nurse's attention to the extreme variation there is not unfrequently in the pulse of such patients during the day. A very common case is this: Between 3 and 4 A.M. the pulse becomes quick, perhaps 130, and so thready it is not like a pulse at all, but like a string vibrating just underneath the skin. After this the patient gets no more sleep. About mid-day the pulse has come down to 80; and though feeble and compressible is a very respectable pulse. At night, if the patient has had a day of excitement, it is almost imperceptible. But, if the patient has had a good day, it is stronger and steadier and not quicker than at mid-day. This is a common history of a common pulse; and others, equally varying during the day, might be given. Now, in inflammation, which may almost always be detected by the pulse, in typhoid fever, which is accompanied by the low pulse that nothing will raise, there is no such great variation. And doctors and nurses become accustomed not to look for it. The doctor indeed cannot. But the variation is in itself an important feature.

Cases like the above often "go off rather suddenly," as it is called, from some trifling ailment of a few days, which just makes up the sum of exhaustion necessary to produce death. And everybody cries, who would have thought it? except the observing nurse, if there is one, who had always expected the exhaustion to come, from which there would be no rally, because she knew the patient had no capital in strength on which to draw, if he failed for a few days to make his barely daily income in sleep and nutrition.

I have often seen really good nurses distressed, because they could not impress the doctor with the real danger of their patient; and quite provoked because the patient "would look," either "so much better" or "so much worse" than he really is "when the doctor was there." The distress is very legitimate, but it generally arises from the nurse not having the power of laying clearly and shortly before the doctor the facts from which she derives her opinion, or from the doctor being hasty and inexperienced, and not capable of eliciting them. A man who really cares for his patients, will soon learn to ask for and appreciate the information of a nurse, who is at once a careful observer and a clear reporter.

house, will be the excess of mortality, that is, the person will die
who ought not to have died before old age.

Now, would it not very materially alter the opinion of whoever
were endeavouring to form one, if he knew that from that floor, of
that house, of that street the man came?

Much more precise might be our observations even than this and
much more correct our conclusions.

It is well known that the same names may be seen constantly
recurring on workhouse books for generations.   That is, the persons
were born and brought up, and will be born and brought up, generation after generation, in the conditions which make paupers.   Death
and disease are like the workhouse, they take from the same family,
the same house, or in other words the same conditions.   Why will
we not observe what they are?

The close observer may safely predict that such a family, whether
its members marry or not, will become extinct; that such another
will degenerate morally and physically.   But who learns the lesson?
On the contrary, it may be well known that the children die in such
a house at the rate of 8 out of 10; one would think that nothing
more need be said; for how could Providence speak more distinctly?
yet nobody listens, the family goes on living there till it dies out,
and then some other family takes it.   Neither would they listen " if
one rose from the dead."

What observa-
tion is for.
In dwelling upon the vital importance of *sound* observation, it
must never be lost sight of what observation is for.   It is not for the
sake of piling up miscellaneous information or curious facts, but for
the sake of saving life and increasing health and comfort.   The
caution may seem useless, but it is quite surprising how many
men (some women do it too), practically behave as if the scientific
end were the only one in view, or as if the sick body were but a
reservoir for stowing medicines into, and the surgical disease
only a curious case the sufferer has made for the attendant's
special information.   This is really no exaggeration.   You think,
if you suspected your patient was being poisoned, say, by a copper
kettle, you would instantly, as you ought, cut off all possible
connection between him and the suspected source of injury, without regard to the fact that a curious mine of observation is
thereby lost.   But it is not everybody who does so, and it has
actually been made a question of medical ethics, what should the
medical man do if he suspected poisoning?   The answer seems a very
simple one,—insist on a confidential nurse being placed with the
patient, or give up the case.

What a con-
fidential nurse
should be.
And remember every nurse should be one who is to be
depended upon, in other words, capable of being a " confidential "
nurse.   She does not know how soon she may find herself placed
in such a situation; she must be no gossip, no vain talker; she
should never answer questions about her sick except to those who
have a right to ask them; she must, I need not say, be strictly
sober and honest; but more than this, she must be a religious
and devoted woman; she must have a respect for her own calling,

because God's precious gift of life is often literally placed in her hands; she must be a sound, and close, and quick observer; and she must be a woman of delicate and decent feeling.

To return to the question of what observation is for:—It would really seem as if some had considered it as its own end, as if detection, not cure, was their business; nay more, in a recent celebrated trial, three medical men, according to their own account, suspected poison, prescribed for dysentery, and left the patient to the poisoner. This is an extreme case. But in a small way, the same manner of acting falls under the cognizance of us all. How often the attendants of a case have stated that they knew perfectly well that the patient could not get well in such an air, in such a room, or under such circumstances, yet have gone on dosing him with medicine, and making no effort to remove the poison from him, or him from the poison which they knew was killing him; nay, more, have sometimes not so much as mentioned their conviction in the right quarter —that is, to the only person who could act in the matter. *Observation is for practical purposes.*

CONCLUSION.

The whole of the preceding remarks apply even more to children and to puerperal women than to patients in general. They also apply to the nursing of surgical, quite as much as to that of medical cases. Indeed, if it be possible, cases of external injury require such care even more than sick. In surgical wards, one duty of every nurse certainly is *prevention*. Fever, or hospital gangrene, or pyœmia, or purulent discharge of some kind may else supervene. Has she a case of compound fracture, of amputation, or of erysipelas, it may depend very much on how she looks upon the things enumerated in these notes, whether one or other of these hospital diseases attacks her patient or not. If she allows her ward to become filled with the peculiar close fœtid smell, so apt to be produced among surgical cases, especially where there is great suppuration and discharge, she may see a vigorous patient in the prime of life gradually sink and die where, according to all human probability, he ought to have recovered. The surgical nurse must be ever on the watch, ever on her guard, against want of cleanliness, foul air, want of light, and of warmth. *Sanitary nursing as essential in surgical as in medical cases, but not to supersede surgical nursing.*

Nevertheless let no one think that because *sanitary* nursing is the subject of these notes, therefore, what may be called the handicraft of nursing is to be undervalued. A patient may be left to bleed to death in a sanitary palace. Another who cannot move himself may die of bed-sores, because the nurse does not know how to change and clean him, while he has every requisite of air, light, and quiet. But nursing, as a handicraft, has not been treated of here for three reasons : 1. that these notes do not pretend to be a manual for nursing, any more than for cooking for the sick; 2. that the writer, who has herself seen more of what may be called surgical nursing, *i. e*, practical manual nursing, than, perhaps, any one in Europe,

honestly believes that it is impossible to learn it from any book, and
that it can only be thoroughly learnt in the wards of a hospital; and
she also honestly believes that the perfection of surgical nursing may
be seen practised by the old-fashioned "Sister" of a London hospital,
as it can be seen nowhere else in Europe. 3. While thousands die
of foul air, &c., who have this surgical nursing to perfection, the
converse is comparatively rare.

**Children :
their greater
susceptibility
to the same
things.**
To revert to children. They are much more susceptible than grown
people to all noxious influences. They are affected by the same
things, but much more quickly and seriously, viz., by want of fresh
air, of proper warmth, want of cleanliness in house, clothes, bedding,
or body, by startling noises, improper food, or want of punctuality,
by dulness and by want of light, by too much or too little covering
in bed, or when up, by want of the spirit of management generally
in those in charge of them. One can, therefore, only press the importance, as being yet greater in the case of children, greatest in the
case of sick children, of attending to these things.

That which, however, above all, is known to injure children
seriously is foul air, and most seriously at night. Keeping the rooms
where they sleep tight shut up, is destruction to them. And, if the
child's breathing be disordered by disease, a few hours only of such
foul air may endanger its life, even where no inconvenience is felt
by grown-up persons in the same room.

The following passages, taken out of an excellent "Lecture on
Sudden Death in Infancy and Childhood," just published, show the
vital importance of careful nursing of children. "In the great
majority of instances, when death suddenly befalls the infant or young
child, it is an *accident;* it is not a necessary, inevitable result of any
disease from which it is suffering."

It may be here added, that it would be very desirable to know
how often death is, with adults, "not a necessary, inevitable result
of any disease." Omit the word "sudden;" (for *sudden* death is
comparatively rare in middle age ;) and the sentence is almost equally
true for all ages.

The following causes of "accidental" death in sick children are
enumerated :—"Sudden noises, which startle—a rapid change of
temperature, which chills the surface, though only for a moment
—a rude awakening from sleep—or even an over-hasty, or an over-
full meal"—" any sudden impression on the nervous system—any
hasty alteration of posture—in short, any cause whatever by which
the respiratory process may be disturbed."

It may again be added, that, with very weak adult patients, these
causes are also (not often "suddenly fatal," it is true, but) very much
oftener than is at all generally known, irreparable in their consequences.

Both for children and for adults, both for sick and for well
(although more certainly in the case of sick children than in any
others), I would here again repeat, the most frequent and most
fatal cause of all is sleeping, for even a few hours, much more for
weeks and months, in foul air, a condition which, more than any

other condition, disturbs the respiratory process, and tends to produce " accidental" death in disease.

I need hardly here repeat the warning against any confusion of ideas between cold and fresh air. You may chill a patient fatally without giving him fresh air at all. And you can quite well, nay, much better, give him fresh air without chilling him. This is the test of a good nurse.

In cases of long recurring faintnesses from disease, for instance, especially disease which affects the organs of breathing, fresh air to the lungs, warmth to the surface, and often (as soon as the patient can swallow) hot drink, these are the right remedies and the only ones. Yet, oftener than not, you see the nurse or mother just reversing this; shutting up every cranny through which fresh air can enter, and leaving the body cold, or perhaps throwing a greater weight of clothes upon it, when already it is generating too little heat.

" Breathing carefully, anxiously, as though respiration were a function which required all the attention for its performance," is cited as a not unusual state in children, and as one calling for care in all the things enumerated above. That breathing becomes an almost voluntary act, even in grown up patients who are very weak, must often have been remarked.

" Disease having interfered with the perfect accomplishment of the respiratory function, some sudden demand for its complete exercise, issues in the sudden stand still of the whole machinery," is given as one process:—" life goes out for want of nervous power to keep the vital functions in activity," is given as another, by which " accidental" death is most often brought to pass in infancy.

Also in middle age, both these processes may be seen ending in death, although generally not suddenly. And I have seen, even in middle age, the " *sudden* stand-still" here mentioned, and from the same causes.

To sum up:—the answer to two of the commonest objections **Summary.** urged, one by women themselves, the other by men, against the desirableness of sanitary knowledge for women, *plus* a caution, comprises the whole argument for the art of nursing.

(1.) It is often said by men, that it is unwise to teach women **Reckless amateur physicking by women.** anything about these laws of health, because they will take to physicking,—that there is a great deal too much of amateur physicking as it is, which is indeed true. One eminent physician told me **Real knowledge of the laws of health alone can check this.** that he had known more calomel given, both at a pinch and for a continuance, by mothers, governesses, and nurses, to children than he had ever heard of a physician prescribing in all his experience. Another says, that women's only idea in medicine is calomel and aperients. This is undeniably too often the case. There is nothing ever seen in any professional practice like the reckless physicking by amateur females.* But this is just what the really experienced and

---

* I have known many ladies who, having once obtained a "blue pill" prescription from a physician, gave and took it as a common aperient two or three times a week—with what effect may be supposed. In one case I happened to be the person to inform the physician of it, who substituted for the prescription a com- **Danger of physicking by amateur females.**

observing nurse does *not* do; she neither physics herself nor others. And to cultivate in things pertaining to health observation and experience in women who are mothers, governesses or nurses, is just the way to do away with amateur physicking, and if the doctors did but know it, to make the nurses obedient to them,—helps to them instead of hindrances. Such education in women would indeed diminish the doctor's work—but no one really believes that doctors wish that there should be more illness, in order to have more work.

What pathology teaches. What observation alone teaches. What medicine does. What nature alone does. (2.) It is often said by women, that they cannot know anything of the laws of health, or what to do to preserve their children's health, because they can know nothing of " Pathology," or cannot " dissect," —a confusion of ideas which it is hard to attempt to disentangle. Pathology teaches the harm that disease has done. But it teaches nothing more. We know nothing of the principle of health, the positive of which pathology is the negative, except from observation and experience. And nothing but observation and experience will teach us the ways to maintain or to bring back the state of health. It is often thought that medicine is the curative process. It is no such thing ; medicine is the surgery of functions, as surgery proper is that of limbs and organs. Neither can do anything but remove obstructions ; neither can cure ; nature alone cures. Surgery removes the

paratively harmless aperient pill. The lady came to me and complained that it " did not suit her half so well."

If women will take or give physic, by far the safest plan is to send for " the doctor" every time—for I have known ladies who both gave and took physic, who would not take the pains to learn the names of the commonest medicines, and confounded, *e. g.*, colocynth with colchicum. This *is* playing with sharp edged tools " with a vengeance."

There are excellent women who will write to London to their physician that there is much sickness in their neighbourhood in the country, and ask for some prescription from him, which they used to like themselves, and then give it to all their friends and to all their poorer neighbours who will take it. Now, instead of giving medicine, of which you cannot possibly know the exact and proper application, nor all its consequences, would it not be better if you were to persuade and help your poorer neighbours to remove the dung-hill from before the door, to put in a window which opens, or an Arnott's ventilator, or to cleanse and lime-wash the cottages ? Of these things the benefits are sure. The benefits of the inexperienced administration of medicines are by no means so sure.

Homœopathy has introduced one essential amelioration in the practice of physic by amateur females ; for its rules are excellent, its physicking comparatively harmless—the "globule" is the one grain of folly which appears to be necessary to make any good thing acceptable. Let then women, if they will give medicine, give homœopathic medicine. It won't do any harm.

An almost universal error among women is the supposition that everybody *must* have the bowels opened once in every twenty-four hours or must fly immediately to aperients. The reverse is the conclusion of experience.

This is a doctor's subject, and I will not enter more into it ; but will simply repeat, do not go on taking or giving to your children your abominable "courses of aperients," without calling in the doctor.

It is very seldom indeed, that by choosing your diet, you cannot regulate your own bowels ; and every woman may watch herself to know what kind of diet will do this ; I have known deficiency of meat produce constipation, quite as often as deficiency of vegetables ; baker's bread much oftener than either. Home made brown bread will oftener cure it than anything else.

bullet out of the limb, which is an obstruction to cure, but nature heals the wound. So it is with medicine; the function of an organ becomes obstructed; medicine, so far as we know, assists nature to remove the obstruction, but does nothing more. And what nursing has to do in either case, is to put the patient in the best condition for nature to act upon him. Generally, just the contrary is done. You think fresh air, and quiet and cleanliness extravagant, perhaps dangerous, luxuries, which should be given to the patient only when quite convenient, and medicine the *sine quâ non*, the panacea. If I have succeeded in any measure in dispelling this illusion, and in showing what true nursing is, and what it is not, my object will have been answered.

Now for the caution :—

(3.) It seems a commonly received idea among men and even among women themselves that it requires nothing but a disappointment in love, the want of an object, a general disgust, or incapacity for other things, to turn a woman into a good nurse.

This reminds one of the parish where a stupid old man was set to be schoolmaster because he was " past keeping the pigs."

Apply the above receipt for making a good nurse to making a good servant. And the receipt will be found to fail.

Yet popular novelists of recent days have invented ladies disappointed in love or fresh out of the drawing-room turning into the war-hospitals to find their wounded lovers, and when found, forthwith abandoning their sick-ward for their lover, as might be expected. Yet in the estimation of the authors, these ladies were none the worse for that, but on the contrary were heroines of nursing.

What cruel mistakes are sometimes made by benevolent men and women in matters of business about which they can know nothing and think they know a great deal.

The everyday management of a large ward, let alone of a hospital —the knowing what are the laws of life and death for men, and what the laws of health for wards—(and wards are healthy or unhealthy, mainly according to the knowledge or ignorance of the nurse)—are not these matters of sufficient importance and difficulty to require learning by experience and careful inquiry, just as much as any other art? They do not come by inspiration to the lady disappointed in love, nor to the poor workhouse drudge hard up for a livelihood.

And terrible is the injury which has followed to the sick from such wild notions!

In this respect (and why is it so ?), in Roman Catholic countries, both writers and workers are, in theory at least, far before ours. They would never think of such a beginning for a good working Superior or Sister of Charity. And many a Superior has refused to admit a *Postulant* who appeared to have no better "vocation " or reasons for offering herself than these.

It is true *we* make "no vows." But is a "vow" necessary to convince us that the true spirit for learning any art, most especially an art of charity, aright, is not a disgust to everything or something else? Do we really place the love of our kind (and of nursing, as one branch of it,) so low as this? What would the Mère Angélique of Port Royal, what would our own Mrs. Fry have said to this?

NOTE.—I would earnestly ask my sisters to keep clear of both the jargons now current everywhere (for they *are* equally jargons); of the jargon, namely, about the "rights" of women, which urges women to do all that men do, including the medical and other professions, merely because men do it, and without regard to whether this *is* the best that women can do; and of the jargon which urges women to do nothing that men do, merely because they are women, and should be "recalled to a sense of their duty as women," and because "this is women's work," and "that is men's," and "these are things which women should not do," which is all assertion and nothing more. Surely woman should bring the best she has, *whatever* that is, to the work of God's world, without attending to either of these cries. For what are they, both of them, the one *just* as much as the other, but listening to the "what people will say," to opinion, to the "voices from without?" And as a wise man has said, no one has ever done anything great or useful by listening to the voices from without.

You do not want the effect of your good things to be, "How wonderful for a *woman!*" nor would you be deterred from good things, by hearing it said, "Yes, but she ought not to have done this, because it is not suitable for a woman." But you want to do the thing that is good, whether it is "suitable for a woman" or not.

It does not make a thing good, that it is remarkable that a woman should have been able to do it. Neither does it make a thing bad, which would have been good had a man done it, that it has been done by a woman.

Oh, leave these jargons, and go your way straight to God's work, in simplicity and singleness of heart.

APPENDIX.

TABLE A.
GREAT BRITAIN.
AGES.

NURSES.	All Ages.	Under 5 Years.	5—	10—	15—	20—	25—	30—	35—	40—	45—	50—	55—	60—	65—	70—	75—	80—	85 and Upwards
Nurse (not Domestic Servant)	25,466	...	...	...	...	624	817	1,118	1,359	2,223	2,748	3,982	3,456	3,825	2,542	1,568	746	311	147
Nurse (Domestic Servant) ...	39,139	...	508	7,259	10,355	6,537	4,174	2,495	1,681	1,468	1,206	1,196	833	712	369	204	101	25	16

TABLE B.
AGED 20 YEARS OF AGE, AND UPWARDS.

	Great Britain and Islands in the British Seas.	England and Wales.	Scotland.	Islands in the British Seas.	1st Division. London.	2nd Division. South Eastern.	3rd Division. South Midland.	4th Division. Eastern Counties.	5th Division. South Western Countrs.	6th Division. West Midland Counties.	7th Division. North Midland Counties.	8th Division. North Western Counties.	9th Division. Yorkshire.	10th Division. Northern Counties.	11th Division. Monmouth, and Wales.
Nurse (not Domestic Servant)	25,466	23,751	1,543	172	7,807	2,878	2,286	2,408	3,055	1,225	1,003	970	1,074	402	343
Nurse (Domestic Servant) ...	21,017	18,915	1,922	150	5,061	2,514	1,252	939	1,737	2,283	957	2,135	1,023	410	614

Note as to the Number of Women employed as Nurses in Great Britain.

25,466 were returned, at the census of 1851, as nurses by profession, 39,139 nurses in domestic service,* and 2,822 midwives. The numbers of different ages are shown in table A, and in table B their distribution over Great Britain.

To increase the efficiency of this class, and to make as many of them as possible the disciples of the true doctrines of health, would be a great national work.

For there the material exists, and will be used for nursing, whether the real " conclusion of the matter" be to nurse or to poison the sick. A man, who stands perhaps at the head of our medical profession, once said to me, I send a nurse into a private family to nurse the sick, but I know that it is only to do them harm.

Now a nurse means any person in charge of the personal health of another. And, in the preceding notes, the term *nurse* is used indiscriminately for amateur and professional nurses. For, besides nurses of the sick and nurses of children, the numbers of whom are here given, there are friends or relations who take temporary charge of a sick person, there are mothers of families. It appears as if these unprofessional nurses were just as much in want of knowledge of the laws of health as professional ones.

Then there are the school-mistresses of all national and other schools throughout the kingdom. How many of children's epidemics originate in these! Then the proportion of girls in these schools, who become mothers or members among the 64,600 nurses recorded above, or schoolmistresses in their turn. If the laws of health, as far as regards fresh air, cleanliness, light, &c., were taught to these, would this not prevent some children being killed, some evil being perpetuated? On women we must depend, first and last, for personal and household hygiene—for preventing the race from degenerating in as far as these things are concerned. Would not the true way of infusing the art of preserving its own health into the human race be to teach the female part of it in schools and hospitals, both by practical teaching and by simple experiments, in as far as these illustrate what may be called the theory of it?

* A curious fact will be shown by Table A, viz., that 18,122 out of 39,139, or nearly one-half of all the nurses, in domestic service, are between 5 and 20 years of age.

A SUMMER SEARCH FOR SIR JOHN FRANKLIN, with a Peep into the Polar Basin, by Commander E. A. Inglefield, R.N. Demy 8vo., 14s.

FRENCH NAVAL TACTICS; Translated from the French by Augustus Phillimore, Captain, R.N. Demy 8vo., 10s.

DESPATCHES AND PAPERS RELATIVE TO CAMpaign in Turkey, Asia Minor, and the Crimea in 1854-5-6, by Captain Sayer.

DESPATCHES OF VISCOUNT HARDINGE, LORD Gough, and Sir Harry Smith. Demy 8vo., 6s.

PRESENT STATE OF THE TURKISH EMPIRE, by Marshal Marmont, translated by General Sir F. Smith, K.H., F.R.S. Second Edition, post 8vo., 7s. 6d.

PASTORAL AND OTHER POEMS, by Mrs. George Halse, Fcap. 8vo., 2s. 6d. cloth.

THE LAUREL AND THE PALM, by Mrs. Challice, Cloth, 6s.

EDA MORTON AND HER COUSINS. Fcap. 8vo., 6s.

CAVENDISH, OR THE PATRICIAN AT SEA, by W. Johnson Neale. Fcap. 8vo., cloth. 2s. 6d.

CHOLLERTON, A TALE OF OUR OWN TIMES, Fcap. 8vo., 7s. 6d.

EVELINA, by Miss Burney. Fcap. 8vo., 3s.

HARRISON, 59, PALL MALL, LONDON, S.W.,
Bookseller to the Queen.

THE PARISH CHOIR, OR CHURCH MUSIC BOOK,
In 3 vols., 21s. cloth.

A PLAIN TRACT ON SINGING IN PUBLIC WOR-
ship. 1d., or 7s. per 100.

CONVERSATIONS ON THE CHORAL SERVICE, being
an Examination of popular prejudices against Church Music. Fcap. 8vo., 1s.

BISHOP BLOMFIELD AND HIS TIMES, by the Rev.
G. E. Biber, LL.D. 1 vol., post 8vo , 7s. 6d.

A PLAIN TRACT ON CHURCH ORNAMENTS, 1d., or
7s. per 100.

HOW TO STOP AND WHEN TO STOP; Punctuation
reduced to a System. Fcap. 8vo., cloth, 1s.

ANTHEMS FOR PARISH CHOIRS, collected and edited by
the Rev. Sir W. H. Cope, Bart. 1 vol., 4to., 9s.

GERMAN, IN FIFTY LESSONS, by Herr C. A. A. Bran,
Fcap. 8vo., 5s. 6d.

THE TURKISH CAMPAIGNER'S VADE-MECUM OF THE
Ottoman Colloquial Language, by J. W. Redhouse, F.R.A.S. Pocket Edition, 4s.
cloth.

COMPARATIVE GRAMMAR OF THE DRAVIDIAN
or South-Indian Family of Languages, by the Rev. R. Caldwell, B.A. Demy 8vo.,
cloth. 21s.

HARRISON, 59, PALL MALL, LONDON, S.W.,
Bookseller to the Queen.

EASY ANTHEMS.

For Four Voices, with Organ or Piano Forte Accompaniments.

O love the Lord	Goldwin	2d.	Deliver us, O Lord our God..	Batten	} 4d.
Praise the Lord	Okeland	2d.	Teach me, O Lord ..	Rogers	
For unto us a Child is Born..	Haselton	2d.	O Praise the Lord ..	Weldon	2d.
O Praise God in his Holiness	Weldon	2d.	Veni, Creator Spiritus ..	Tallis	3d.
Behold, now Praise the Lord	Rogers	2d.	Out of the Deep	Aldrich	6d.

The above ANTHEMS, forming PART I, may also be had in Wrapper, 2s.

O Praise the Lord ..	Batten	2d.	O How Amiable	Richardson	} 3d.
Plead Thou my Cause	Glareanus	2d.	Offertory Anthem ..	Whitbroke	
Praise the Lord, O Jerusalem	Scott	4d.	Not unto Us, O Lord	Aldrich	3d.
My Soul Truly Waiteth	Batten	2d.	Hear my Prayer ..	Batten	4d.
If Ye Love Me	Tallis	2d.	Lord, Who shall dwell	Rogers	4d.
Thou Visitest the Earth	Greene	2d.			

The above ANTHEMS, forming PART II, may also be had in Wrapper, 2s.

Have mercy upon Me ..	Gibbs	2d.	O Israel, Trust in the Lord ..	Croft	2d.
Wherewithal shall a Young Man..	Alcock	2d.	Blessing and Glory	Boyce	2d.
I give you a New Commandment..	Shephard	3d.	Lift Up Your Heads ..	Turner	2d.
Holy, Holy, Holy ..	Bishop	2d.	Thou Knowest, Lord ..	Purcell	} 2d.
Call to Remembrance	Farrant	2d.	Set up Thyself, O God ..	Wise	
Teach Me Thy Way, O Lord	Fox	} 2d.	Behold now, Praise the Lord	Creyghton	2d.
Blessed art Thou, O Lord	Weldon		Gloria in Excelsis ..	S. Mark's use	2d.

The above ANTHEMS, forming PART III, may also be had in Wrapper, 2s.

The Three Parts, forming Vol. I of EASY ANTHEMS, may be had, neatly bound together in cloth, price 6s.

O Praise the Lord ..	Goldwin	2d.	O Lord, Grant the King	Child	
O Give Thanks	Rogers	} 4d.	Behold How Good and Joyful	Rogers	2d.
Lord, We Beseech Thee	Batten		The Lord is King ..	King	2d.
Offertory Anthems..	Monk	2d.	Sing We Merrily ..	Batten	4d.
Glory be to God on High	Loosemore	4d.	O Pray for the Peace ..	Rogers	4d.
Lord, for Thy Tender Mercies	Farrant	2d.			

The above ANTHEMS, forming PART IV, may also be had in Wrapper, 2s.

ANTHEMS FOR PARISH CHOIRS,

By Eminent Composers of the English Church.

Collected and Edited by the Rev. SIR WILLIAM H. COPE, Bart., Minor Canon of St. Peter's, Westminster.

No. I. (Price 8d.) Contains:

Sing we merrily	Adrian Batten
Let my complaint	Ditto
I will not leave you comfortless	Dr. William Byrde

No. II. (Price 10d.) Contains:

O Clap your hands ..	Dr. William Child
When the Lord turned again ..	Adrian Batten
O Pray for the Peace of Jerusalem	Dr. Benj. Rogers
How long wilt Thou forget me ..	Ditto

No. III. (Price 1s.) Contains:

Oh! that the salvation ..	Dr. Benj. Rogers
Praise the Lord, O my soul ..	Ditto
O Give thanks unto the Lord..	Ditto
Save me; O God	Ditto
Behold how good and joyful ..	Ditto

No. IV. (Price 8d.) Contains:

By the waters of Babylon	Rev. Dr. H. Aldrich
Not unto us, O Lord	Thomas Kelway
O praise the Lord all ye heathen	John Goldwin

No. V. (Price 8d.) Contains:

Haste Thee, O God, to deliver me	Adrian Batten
Why art thou so heavy ..	Dr. Orlando Gibbons
Behold now praise the Lord ..	Rev. Dr. H. Aldrich

No. VI. (Price 10d.) Contains:

Praise the Lord, O my soul ..	Dr. John Blow
In Thee, O Lord, have I put my trust	William Evans

No. VII. (Price 8d.) Contains:

Unto Thee O Lord, will I lift up ..	Thomas Kelway
The Lord is King ..	William King
In the beginning, O Lord	Matthew Lock

No. VIII. (Price 1s.) Contains:

Let God arise ..	Matthew Lock
Sing unto the Lord a new song	Ditto
When the Son of Man shall come	Ditto
Lord, we beseech Thee ..	Adrian Batten

No. IX. (Price 8d.) Contains:

O Lord, I have loved the habitation	Thomas Tomkins
Great and marvellous ..	Ditto
He that hath pity upon the poor	Ditto

No. X. (Price 10d.) Contains:

O Lord God of our salvation ..	Rev. Dr. H. Aldrich
Lord, who shall dwell ..	Adrian Batten
O Praise the Lord : laud ye ..	Dr. William Child

ISBN 0-397-55007-3

90000

9 780397 550074